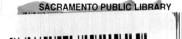

What People are Saying about *UnBr*

"*UnBreak Your Health* is the most comprehensive and reader-friendly guide for alternative health solutions that I have ever read. The author, Alan E. Smith, through personal experience presents a compelling argument for the power of our bodies to heal themselves if we would give them the opportunity. The methods listed in this book include therapies that have been around for thousands of years to new life-changing devices. *UnBreak Your Health* would complement any home-based or business library. I applaud the author for creating such a comprehensive guide."

—Reviewed by Cherie Fisher for *Reader Views*

"*UnBreak Your Health: The Complete Guide to Complementary & Alternative Therapies* is a good overview of a number of different types of holistic mind/body/spirit healing practices."

—Eric Robins, M.D., co-author of *Your Hands Can Heal You*

"I love that it is written in lay language—it is an every person's guide! So many books comparing complementary medicine techniques and medical or health modalities are not; the reader must usually wade through technical terms and small print as if reading a legal contract. Needless to say, many of those truly desiring help are discouraged and explore no more. Alan Smith's book is a welcome and needed addition for those who truly desire access to health and wellness information in easily digestible language and backed up by diverse experiences."

—Imara, MBA, MHpn, URM
TheWisdomLight.com

"There are many ways to heal and many ways to grow. *UnBreak Your Health* offers an amazing and impressive collection of valuable information to people looking to complement the conventional methods of treatment."

—Karen Carnabucci, LCSW, TEP
CompanionsInHealing.com

"*Unbreak Your Health* has a great concept going for it. Alternative health techniques have flooded the market in recent years, and their sheer variety overwhelms most people. It's a laudable goal of Smith's to explain these many practices, which he does clearly and concisely. Smith also covers an amazing number of therapies in a mere 212 pages."

—Reviewed by Elizabeth A. Allen for *Clarion Reviews*

Health Solutions From The Newest Technology to Ancient Therapies

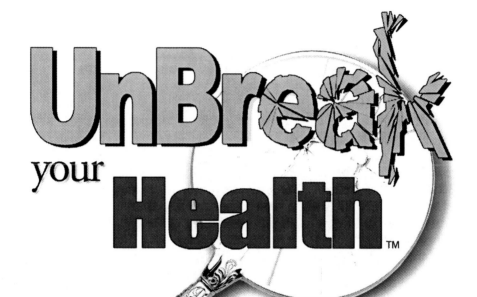

UnBreak
your Health™

*The Complete Guide
to Complementary
& Alternative Therapies*

ALAN E. SMITH

First Edition: October 2007

ISBN-13: 978-1-932690-36-1
ISBN-10: 1-932690-36-0

Library of Congress Cataloging-in-Publication Data

Smith, Alan E., 1951-
     Unbreak your health : the complete guide to complementary & alternative therapies / by Alan E. Smith. -- 1st ed.
          p. cm.
     Includes bibliographical references and index.
     ISBN-13: 978-1-932690-36-1 (trade paper : alk. paper)
     ISBN-10: 1-932690-36-0 (trade paper : alk. paper)
     1. Alternative medicine--Encyclopedias. I. Title.
     R733.S62 2007
     615.5'303--dc22

                                        2007022714

Distributed by:
Quality Books, Ingram Book Group, New Leaf Distributing

Published by:
Loving Healing Press
5145 Pontiac Trail
Ann Arbor, MI 48105
USA

http://www.LovingHealing.com or
info@LovingHealing.com
Fax +1 734 663 6861

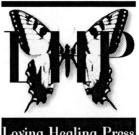

Loving Healing Press

TABLE OF CONTENTS

Disclaimer

This book is not intended to diagnose or prescribe any treatment for any medical or psychological condition(s), nor does it claim to prevent, diagnose, treat, mitigate, or cure any medical or psychological conditions.

It contains the ideas and opinions of its author and is intended solely to provide helpful information on a variety of subjects. It is sold with the understanding that the author and publisher are not engaged in rendering medical, health or any other kind of personal professional services in the book.

The reader should consult his or her medical, health or other competent professional before adopting any of the suggestions in the book.

The author and publisher specifically disclaim all responsibility for any liability, loss, or risk, personal or otherwise, that is incurred as a consequence (directly or indirectly) of the use and application of any of the contents of this book.

Introduction

This book is all about hope. From ancient healing therapies to the latest American innovations, you have more options for great health today than ever before. Complementary and alternative therapies, known as CAM, are about more than just improving your health. These therapies are about helping you rediscover the joy, the wonder and the beauty of living.

They say you can't "unbreak the mirror", meaning the damage is done. In the world of healthcare the analogy would be mainstream medicine treating the symptoms of the broken mirror with drugs to try and glue it back together. To *UnBreak Your Health*™ means discovering the real source of the problem and treating all of it. What happened that caused you to drop the mirror in the first place? Perhaps the aches and pains that caused you to stumble are caused from your body being out of alignment in some way so it's a body issue. Maybe an emotional issue or traumatic life experience is seeking resolution by expressing itself through the body, so it could be a mind issue. Or your life force energy could be blocked in some way resulting in a physical problem so it could be a spirit or energy issue.

In this guide you'll also discover incredible new devices like a top-secret Russian military technology used in their space program (*SKENAR*). You'll find out about Dr. Bjorn Nordenstrom's discovery of an energy circulation system in the human body (see *Energy Medicine*), remarkably similar to ancient Chinese concepts (see *Traditional Chinese Medicine*). Doctors in the U.S. have said this could be the most important medical discovery in 350 years. You'll find information new and old and begin to see patterns and concepts between therapies that are consistent through thousands of years and across civilizations around the world.

The most basic concept is that you are the sum of your Mind-Body-Spirit and therefore a problem in one area can mean problems in all areas. Holistic (or whole-istic) therapies can be so effective because they address all of you. You're about to discover how complementary and alternative therapies work to prevent problems or correct them as soon as possible to prevent them from growing into serious issues.

Once you start talking with friends and family about these options, it seems like everybody knows somebody who's experienced success, sometimes miraculous success, with a complementary or alternative therapy. While writing this book, I've been amazed at the stories from friends and yet we still seem to talk about CAM in whispers, as if it's something normal people didn't discuss in public. I hope this book brings complementary and alternative therapies out of the shadows and into the light of day so more people can discover a healthier, happier new life.

The majority of Americans (62%) have already used some form of complementary and alternative therapy during the previous 12 months, according to a 2002 federal government report. This data is from the National Health Interview Survey conducted by the U. S. Department of Health & Human Services, the Center for Disease Control's National Center for Health Statistics. The growth of CAM in the past twenty years has been phenomenal, especially considering that the majority of the billions of dollars spent have been by individuals, not the government or insurance companies.

Perhaps one of the reasons for the explosive growth and popularity of complementary and alternative therapies is the appreciation of a person as much more than just a number on a form. Every person is a unique individual composed of mind, body and spirit (or life-force energy). All facets must be healthy and balanced for wellness and personal growth. A PBS-TV special in 2006 featured doctors talking about their hope for the trend in medicine to go back to treating patients as whole beings. Many of them wondered how Western medicine could have ever gotten so far off track to ignore the mind and spiritual components of every patient in the first place.

Complementary and alternative therapies also focus on individualized treatments, rather than assembly-line medicine. Every person and their health problems are unique, usually resulting from a combination of factors. These therapies tend to look at the whole person for the source of the problem, not just the symptoms that bring them in the door.

In this era of entitlement, too many people have come to believe they are owed good health and this has led to a passive national attitude towards health. When we get sick, we expect the doctor to give us a pill, a shot or perform some surgery to fix us right up so we can continue living without having to make any changes. One of the major themes of complementary and alternative therapies is personal responsibility. Who better to take care of *your* body than YOU? These complementary and alternative therapies offer new and old ways for better health but you, the person reading this book, will have to care enough about living to take personal responsibility for your life.

Another difference between standard medicine and CAM today is a focus on wellness and the ingredients for health. Among other things, we need proper diet, exercise and a way to release the stress of the day. You've probably already heard these recommendations from medical doctors. These aren't new ideas; in fact they're very old. Hundreds of years ago Johnathan Swift, author of *Gulliver's Travels*, said that "The best doctors in the world are Doctor Diet, Doctor Quiet and Doctor Merryman." Today, we usually take better care of our cars and our yards than we do our most precious gift, our own health.

America has neglected complementary and alternative therapies in favor of scientific Western medicine for over 100 years. While this profit-driven orientation has produced some outstanding developments, much has also been sacrificed. Today, the newest equipment is confirming that we are all *whole beings* of mind, body and spirit, often raising more questions than providing answers. The explosion of research in neuroscience is changing the meaning of the expression "It's all in your head" because technology is showing how the mind is related to and controls the body. We're moving quickly from simply correlation of the mind-body connection to discovering the actual mechanisms of interaction.

Changes have already slowly begun to take place in mainstream medicine. The National Institutes of Health conducted a survey in 2005 reporting nearly 27% of those hospitals responding were offering one or more CAM therapies. The most popular CAM in-patient therapy being offered was massage with a 37% response rate. Music and Art Therapy was the second most common in-patient therapy offered at 26%.

You've probably heard many opinions about the Placebo Effect and I'll take this opportunity to add another one up front. I believe the Placebo Effect is simply the body's natural ability to heal itself of everything from the common cold to cancer. The process has no side effects, is non-toxic, and is completely natural and safe. It may, in fact, be the benchmark for the body's natural healing ability. Trying to rush it beyond its natural design may be causing problems.

Because so many of these complementary and alternative therapies are based on a completely different paradigm (energy) they operate on different principles than the standard chemical model of the human body. This means they can't be studied using the same methodology as current research. They also function as whole systems and cannot be examined piece by piece. Using existing research models for CAM is simply like trying to put a square peg in a round hole. Much like quantum physics, the very act of observation influences the results. Even the White House Commission on Complementary and Alternative Medicine Policy understood this concept. The 2002 report said "Research is needed to pursue answers to questions posed by CAM that lie outside the conventional medical paradigm."

Everything in this book will work for someone, but nothing in this book will work for everyone. The same is true with mainstream medicine. Some pills help people while the same medication may be ineffective or even harmful to someone else. There is a wide variety and quality of medical doctors and of the practitioners of these healing arts. Whether it's a medical doctor or an alternative practitioner you should always research their qualifications and training and then enter into any relationship with an attitude of Buyer Beware. Remember, you are in charge of your health! Just as it's always been recommended to seek out second opinions for diagnosis by a medical doctor, practicing the same approach would be beneficial when working with complementary or alternative therapies too.

Not every type of CAM will be found in this book. Quite frankly, some are practiced by only a few people while others are being created so quickly that it's almost impossible to keep track. Being human, it's possible my research has missed some valuable therapies too. Some of the therapies listed are FDA approved but because they're still ignored by most doctors, they're still considered outside of the "norm". A list of resources is included at the end of this book for continuing research in new developments and contrary opinions.

What started out as a quest to improve my own Baby Boomer health has resulted in this collection of information and opportunities. Like so many people, conventional medicine ran out of ideas to help me, so I had to start looking for new options, fortunately I've found them. Researching this book has been an enjoyable and enlightening adventure.

This reference guide to complementary and alternative therapies is the result of research and interpretation of each modality, or type of process. In many cases there are a variety of opinions, so please remember this is simply *one* opinion. With the steady stream of innovation happening today this volume is not intended as a finished work but simply a starting place for your quest for better health and a better life.

How to Use This Book

You're probably hoping for a nice American-style book where you can just look up your condition or disease and find all of the complementary and alternative therapies for it. Sorry, but that's not how most CAM therapies work, and it's not how this book works either. This is a place to begin your journey to health and happiness, not a quick fix, so reading this whole book will be the first stop in taking responsibility for your life. Learning about all of these opportunities will give you a better understanding about what's available today.

Do you remember the old joke about the three blind mice and the elephant? One is holding on to the tail and he says "An elephant is long and skinny with hair on the end." The next mouse is touching the leg and he says, "No, an elephant is big and round." The third mouse is on the trunk and he says, "You're both wrong. It's not too thick or too thin, but watch out for all of the hot air!" It's similar when you're trying to figure out what's causing your pain or problem; you need to look at your whole being for the source, rather than just the individual symptoms.

Just because you may have a name for your condition doesn't mean it's the source of your problem, you have to see the whole elephant. Let me give you an example: let's say you have a pain in your shoulder, so you go to your friendly medical doctor. He checks it out and finds there is nothing broken or torn so he gives you a drug for pain, maybe one for muscle relaxation and possibly another drug to reduce inflammation. (Remember Vioxx?)

A practitioner of a complimentary or alternative therapy is usually going to look at you as a whole system to see what's causing the problem. Perhaps you're moving the shoulder in an awkward manner which is causing the strain and pain. A Rolfer or Feldenkrais practitioner is going to realign your body so it moves correctly, removing the strain which eliminates the pain without drugs.

Or perhaps there is a problem with an organ or body function that has changed your body's energy system causing the muscles to tighten in an unusual way which puts a strain on the body. A therapy like acupuncture would realign your body's energy flow and repair the problem.

The Alexander Method would have taught you how to move with efficiency to prevent the wear and tear in the first place. Or perhaps it's stress that's literally beating you down and putting your body into awkward positions. Tai Chi, yoga or meditation would help relieve the stress before it results in a physical problem. (By the way, some doctors now say that up to 80% of our physical problems could actually be stress-related.)

This is just an example of how CAM therapies treat the source of the problem, not just the symptoms. Practitioners of complementary and alternative therapies look at the whole person to find what's wrong so they can correct the problem where it begins, rather than where it ends.

First, let's look at how these complimentary and alternative therapies relate to Western medicine. Today the accepted definition of "integrative medicine" describes it as beginning with the conventional mainstream medical process but also including other healing methods like herbal preparations, biofeedback, acupuncture and other types of CAM therapy as needed.

The term "complementary medicine" is understood to be all other systems of treatment which can complement conventional therapies. An "alternative therapy" is considered a stand-alone option disconnected from standard Western medicine. Another benefit to reading this book is that you can learn how the same CAM therapy may be used in different ways, or how different therapy combinations can work with traditional medicine. While one mainstream doctor may consider a particular therapy a complementary one, another doctor who lacks familiarity may consider it alternative at best. Almost the same situation continues to exist in mainstream medicine about techniques already considered to be part of mainstream medicine.

This book organizes these therapies into three categories: Body, Mind and Energy/Spirit. After careful consideration, each subject is classified based on my opinion regarding the primary goal or operating principle.

For example, Energy Medicine can be found in the Health Concepts section. This subject is based on the incredible discovery by Dr. Bjorn Nordenstrom of a new circulatory system in the human body for electrical energy called the Biological Closed Energy Circuit (BCEC). Since it deals with the physical system of moving energy through the body it's classified as a physical subject although it deals with the body's energy.

Acupuncture, on the other hand, is classified in the Energy/Spirit section even though it also deals with the body's energy system. Because it was developed 5,000 years ago the ancient Chinese called it chi, or life force. They described it as being a balance of Yin and Yang forces in the body, while Dr. Nordenstrom calls it positive and negative electrical energy. These two listings may, in fact, be talking about the same system but they're classified into two different categories based upon their focus.

In an effort to help understand each subject as well as possible similarities to other therapies I often include a little history or perspective with a description of each listing. As you read through this book you'll begin to see many common features and concepts.

User Comments have been included at the end of many listings for a better understanding of each therapy. These are anonymous comments from people who've actually experienced each process. Comments from different people are found in separate paragraphs. These testimonials have been collected from a variety of sources to give you a more personal perspective on each therapy. Please remember results are unique to each individual. Because of our uniqueness a process that works well for one person may perform very differently for another. This feature will at least provide a little human color to the black-and-white definitions and descriptions.

Most listings offer websites for you to begin your own research into selected processes. While many websites are available, remember these are just one place to begin your own process of exploration.

Please read this book with an open mind interested in the big picture, not just to find a magic bullet answer to your current health issues. All of this information will filter deep into your mind and you'll discover that you're naturally drawn to certain subjects. You'll want to reread certain sections over and over, and you'll want to learn more. You'll be happy you did! It's likely your subconscious mind or Higher Self is trying to point your life in the right direction. Just as I've discovered new ways to health, so can you.

Chapter 1 – Health Concepts

AMERICAN PSYCHOSOMATIC SOCIETY

www.psychosomatic.org/

The **American Psychosomatic Society** is one of the major organizations involved in understanding the relationship between mind, body and spirit. It was founded in 1942 for the scientific understanding of the whole human system and promoting improved health. The original effort was to assemble the psychosomatic medical literature to examine the relationship of religion to health. Their first volume was *Emotions and Bodily Changes* published in 1935.

Also called Mind-Body Science, it is the focal point for research into the mind-body connection. In a March 2006 article in the *Wall Street Journal* entitled "All In Your Head? Yes, and Scientists Are Figuring Out Why," association president, Richard Lane said "With the explosion in neuroscience, mind-body medicine can now bring the brain in. That holds out the possibility of moving from correlation to mechanism" showing how the mind is related to the body.

The article went on to explain that everyone is aware at an almost instinctive level that how you think and feel affects your body but because scientists haven't found the mechanisms, the medical community hasn't taken the concept seriously. New research offers brain-based explanations which give greater credibility to the concept so doctors will be more likely to recognize the importance of the mind to the health of the body.

ANTHROPOSOPHICALLY EXTENDED MEDICINE (AEM)

www.artemisia.net

Anthroposophically Extended Medicine was developed by Rudolf Steiner and Ita Wegman, M.D. as a holistic approach to medicine. The name describes the fact that all practitioners must first be licensed medical doctors before taking additional training in therapy, alchemy and the spiritual scientific studies outlined by Rudolf Steiner. While it recognizes the accomplishments of Western medicine, it goes further by adding knowledge in the areas of the psyche and spiritual. The synergy from this combination provides for an integrated view of the human being as a living organism.

There are four integrated parts in each human being. First is the Physical Body which is the focus of Western medicine. The second part is called the Etheric Body, which is the higher power that directs the body's growth and regeneration. The third part is the Astral Body, which is what gives us our instincts and the qualities of our soul. The fourth is the unique human concept of Ego, which gives us the power to shape our own destiny. Together they form a framework for diagnosis and therapy.

The major principles of AEM include that Spirit manifests both within human beings and outside in the substances of nature. That wisdom which created nature also works in people. Every substance or process in nature corresponds directly to the inner workings of man.

Art is an indispensable part of life and artistic therapies can strongly affect the disease processes. Every AEM treatment aims to enhance the life force of the patient. This personal power is the basis for improved health along with deepened self-knowledge.

Mistletoe is an example of the use of natural plants and substances. It has been used as a medicine for cancer patients in Europe since 1917. Patients widely use the prescription product in many countries including Germany. The substance is said to support the immune system and improve the quality of life of cancer patients.

The Anthroposophical Spiritual Science is a fundamental part of this approach. Centuries of this knowledge have been developed by monastics, alchemists, Rosicrucians, Auroleus Phillipus Theostratus Bombastus von Hohenheim (known as "Paracelsus") and Christian Friedrich Samuel Hahnemann (the founder of homeopathic medicine) among others. Out of Anthroposophical Medicine, specialized disciplines of Therapeutic Eurythmy, Rhythmical Massage, clay modeling, painting and music therapy have evolved.

In the U.S., the Physicians' Association for Anthroposophical Medicine was founded in 1981. AEM is a leader in the holistic health movement in Europe. *(Also see listing for Therapeutic Eurythmy.)*

AYURVEDA

www.ayurvedahc.com

Ayurveda in Sanskrit means "The Science of Life" and it's believed to be more than 5,000 years old making it one of the oldest health systems in the world. Developed in India, Ayurvedic medicine focuses on developing a balance of mind, body and spirit to maintain health and prevent illness. Each person is unique, with an individual energy signature, their own mix of physical, mental and emotional characteristics. Proper thinking, lifestyle, diet and herbs are used to achieve proper balance for each person. There are many similarities between Ayurveda and Traditional Chinese Medicine.

The vital energy of a person is called **Prana** which is centered around the energy centers in the body called **Chakras**. Unlike the Chinese system of Yin/Yang, the Indian energy system has three separate elements or doshas:

- **Vata Dosha** – composed of space and air, it is the energy of movement.
- **Patta Dosha** – is made of fire and water, it's the body's metabolic processes.
- **Kapha Dosha** – is the glue that holds it together, the body's structure represented by earth and water.

Ayurveda uses a holistic approach with therapies that appeal to all of the senses to treat each individual. Practitioners may use Taste (herbs and nutrition); Touch (massage, yoga, exercise); Smell (aromatherapy); Sight (color therapy); Hearing (music therapy, mantra meditation, chanting) and Spiritual therapy. The system is about more than health, it's about living.

In many cases, a practitioner will begin by recommending a **Panchakarma** or cleansing process to eliminate the accumulated toxins in the body. **Basti** refers to giving medications rectally to treat **vata dosha**, or problems related to Vata by cleansing the colon. **Nasya** means giving medications nasally and may be either wet or dry. **Virechana** means cleansing of the pitta through the lower pathways.

In the U.S. today, Ayurveda positions itself as a complement to Western medicine, a way to prevent illness by reducing stress and maintaining balance so the body's own defenses can function effectively.

USER COMMENTS: *"This healing system is completely individualized and comprehensive. It's about what type of body you have and the healthiest lifestyle for you. Imbalance in the body leads to disease and malfunction so everything is about maintaining balance. Since I'm a "patta" or fire, I have to cut down on spicy foods in the summer. Ayurveda isn't interested in putting a particular name on a disease, they want to know the cause of the problem. They realize that the same set of symptoms can come from a variety of imbalances depending on each individual, which is why they're so focused on each person. They'll check your tongue, fingernails, all sorts of tests and talk with you about your life and lifestyle to completely learn who you are before trying to determine what the source of the problem really is. Individual differences also make a huge difference in their prescriptions to improve your health depending on your body.*

"This process focuses on the body's normal functions which are so often stymied in America. We have air conditioning so we don't sweat toxins from our body. We go to the bathroom on breaks, not when we want to, frustrating the body's attempt to eliminate waste and toxins in a timely manner which leads to plaque build up in the colon. You can see how it's not hard to let toxins build up to the point that there is a problem.

"There is even balance for the mind and spirit as well since too much media can cause imbalance in that part of your total body system. They believe in a media fast to create balance since many diseases (smoking, alcoholism, etc.) can result from mental imbalances. They also use a head massage with oils to cool the head so the body can function properly. Massage, especially with oils, is a big part of their process because it helps them move toxins around and out of the body."

"These herbs are an organic part of my 'medicine cabinet' and many have gained respect from other Western scientists."

"As a limo driver I never leave my car. I drive and eat in the seat and get no exercise. My stomach was hurting and not digesting any foods. The Fire Harmony has improved my digestion and I get out stretching once in awhile."

"I have been giving my children Water Harmony during the winter months and they are the only ones in their class not to get the flu."

ENERGY MEDICINE (EChT)

www.iabc.readywebsites.com/page/page/623957.htm

The new science of **Energy Medicine** is based on the scientific discovery of a new circulatory system in the human body for electrical energy. This process is remarkably similar to the meridian concepts of Traditional Chinese Medicine.

This new physiologic concept was discovered by internationally renowned Swedish radiologist and surgeon Dr. Bjorn E. W. Nordenstrom and published in *Biologically Closed Electrical Circuits* (1983). Beginning in the mid-1950s Dr. Nordenstrom noticed radiating patterns around cancer tumors on chest X-rays which he called corona structures because they reminded him of the sun's corona. Additional study revealed fluctuating electrical charges within the tumors. This led to the discovery of a new type of system, an electrical circuit that involves the transportation of ions and electrons throughout the body. This circulating current helps maintain the body's equilibrium and healing processes by influencing cellular structure and function.

Blood plasma and interstitial fluid are examples of media capable of conducting current while blood vessel walls, cells and membranes surrounding interstitial spaces provide insulation to the surroundings. In other words, they're insulated electric cables providing communication within the body through electromagnetic signaling. These flowing electrical charges found in the body resemble the "yin and yang" concepts and the flow of Chi discovered 5,000 years ago in ancient China.

The editor of The American Institute of Stress, Paul J. Rosch, M.D., F.A.C.P. wrote in his review of the book that "... he has demonstrated how specific DC microcurrents that restore ion electricity balance can be utilized to treat metastic lung cancer and other malignancies with amazing success, and his therapeutic triumphs have now been replicated by others in thousands of patients." Following a report by Dr. Tim Johnson on ABC's *20/20* program, host Barbara Walters expressed amazement at this medical breakthrough. Thousands of cancer patients around the world have now successfully been treated with electrochemical therapy (EChT) using Dr. Nordenstrom's BCEC concepts.

There are only a few limited trials being conducted in America today. In what may be one of the most fundamental paradigm shifts in medicine since William Harvey discovered blood circulation 350 years ago, America is taking a back seat in research. Unable to secure funding and support in America,

Dr. Nordenstrom was welcomed by China to continue his research. The current five year survival rates for liver cancer are reported to be about 15% in China compared to 5% in the U.S. where they're treated with conventional therapies. In 2001, Dr. Nordenstrom received the International Scientific and Technological Cooperation Award from the People's Republic of China for his work.

EChT treatment is available in Germany, China and other countries. Costs are reported to be in the $7,500 (U.S.) range with treatment taking up to two weeks.

The International Association for Biologically Closed Electric Circuits (BCEC) in Medicine and Biology was founded in 1993 for the development of electrotherapeutic, thermotherapeutic and magnetotherapeutic techniques, along with conventional therapies, for the treatment of health problems including cancer.

ENVIRONMENTAL MEDICINE

Website: www.aaem.com, www.aehf.com. www.niehs.nih.gov

Environmental Medicine is a new perspective and approach that decreases the focus on the disease and increases the awareness of the causes, frequently the environment of the person. It is a comprehensive, proactive, patient-centric approach to medical care dedicated to the management and prevention of environmental problems. In contrast, Western medicine often treats the environment and diet as benign factors in the health equation even though there continues to be explosive growth in the occurrence of more complex and chronic diseases in America.

The new model of environmental medicine employs both Western and Eastern concepts with an appreciation that human beings are constantly coping and adapting to a dynamic environment. **Homeodynamic functioning** refers to the maintenance of health as an active process with optimal health being a balance of physical, neuro-cognitive, psychological and social wellbeing. Stressors to this balance range from organic substances like molds and pollens to man-made chemicals and physical factors like heat, cold, noise and various types of radiation. Treatments for each patient must be customized because each person is a unique organism.

Treatment begins with patient education about the nature of the illness. Therapies may include customized diets, nutritional supplements, immunotherapies, psychotherapies, detoxification therapies, drugs and possibly even surgery.

The American Academy of Environmental Medicine was formed in 1965. It provides the only comprehensive continuing education and training program for MDs and DOs in environmental medicine. The American and International Boards of Environmental Medicine are independent groups which grant board certification and establish educational and training criteria. As with all therapies, it is recommended that customers research and review the training and qualifications of their providers.

HOLISTIC MEDICINE

www.ahha.org, www.holisticmedicine.org

Holistic Medicine is an approach of healing that encompasses the whole person—body, mind and spirit. It involves both conventional and complimentary therapies for greater health and to prevent disease.

Holistic healthcare providers see people as the sum of body, mind, spirit and the systems in which they live. Imbalances in the physical, emotional, spiritual or social environments can result in a loss of health. Healing takes place naturally when these elements are brought into proper balance. Practitioners of Holistic Medicine actively promote health with the goal of preventing illness rather than dealing with symptoms.

Everyone has the power to heal their own body, mind and spirit and the holistic medicine approach is to help patients discover and use these powers. While practitioners believe that love is the most powerful healer in life, they also utilize a variety of resources and approaches to meet the unique needs of each individual. They work with the latest developments of conventional medicine, but they also use options from a variety of healing traditions.

Insurance coverage varies so it is best to discuss your options with your carrier before visiting the holistic doctor's office. In many cases, there is no reimbursement but one option may be for you to increase the amount of deductible in your plan and use the savings for the cost of preventative holistic healthcare. After all, preventing illness and focusing on wellness are the most cost effective form of healthcare in the long run.

The American Holistic Medical Association was created in 1978. Membership is open to medical doctors, doctors of osteopathic medicine and medical students. Board certification in holistic medicine is by certification exam from the American Board of Holistic Medicine.

HOMEOPATHIC MEDICINE or Homeotherapeutics

www.homeopathyusa.org, homeopathic.org

Homeopathy or **homeotherapeutics** is a system of medicine based on the Law of Similars, or "let likes be cured by likes". It takes a holistic perspective of people and illness with the goal of promoting optimal health. According to the World Health Organization, it is the second most practiced form of medicine in the world today. The U.S. survey on complementary and alternative medicine (2002) reported that 1.7% of those questioned said they'd used homeopathy in the prior 12 months and 3.6% said they'd used it at some time in their lives.

In this system, an illness is simply the body's attempt to heal itself and homeopathic remedies trigger the body's self-healing abilities by increasing the life force and correcting imbalances. The process stimulates an accelerated immune system response and releases underlying energetic blocks by using minute amounts of substances that serve as a catalyst to the body. These substances may be from plants, minerals, animals or even from chemical drugs, but they are carefully diluted until very little of the original is left in the solution. All homeopathic medicines are made with the processes described in the official manufacturing manual called the Homeopathic Pharmacopoeia of the United States which is recognized by the FDA.

Homeopathy was first theorized by Hippocrates, but it was German doctor C. F. Samuel Hahnemann who is credited with its first practical application in 1796. It was brought to the U.S. around 1825 by doctors trained in Europe and by 1900 there were an estimated 22 homeopathic medical colleges. Estimates were that 20% of U.S. doctors used homeopathy at that time. However, the move towards the mechanical model of the human body pushed homeopathy out of the main stream.

Homeopathy has been proven to be more effective than mainstream or allopathic medicine in the treatment and prevention of disease without harmful side effects. In a frequently quoted bit of American history, it's reported that the cholera outbreak in 1849 saw allopathic medicine have death rates of 48-60% while homeopathic hospitals had a death rate of only 3%. Today dentists and even veterinarians are increasingly turning to homeopathy. There is also renewed public interest in homeopathy due in some part to the threat of terrorism.

Sequential Homeopathy is a relatively recent development in the field to address multiple blockages or problems. This method uses multiple remedies to reverse the chronological layers causing each problem. Practitioners see clients every 1-2 months because each layer requires 4-8 weeks to release its toxins and heal the affected organs and systems. This process if often used to treat allergies, autism spectrum disorders and auto-immune diseases where the body is attacking itself to recover from toxicity contained in the cells.

The American Institute of Homeopathy was established in 1844 and it remains the oldest national medical profession in the United States. The National Center for Homeopathy has offered instruction in homeopathy for more than 70 years. There are many training programs in homeopathy, but no certificate is recognized as a license to practice homeopathy in this country. Laws regarding homeopathy vary widely from state to state but normally it can be practiced legally by licensed medical professionals. New health freedom laws are increasingly permitting it to be practiced by non-licensed professionals as well so check to see what regulations apply where you live. In addition, homeopathic remedies are sold over the counter for self-care.

NAPRAPATHY

www.naprapathy.us

Naprapathy was developed by Dr. Oakley Smith in 1907 as a treatment process for evaluating and healing damaged connective tissues. The term comes from the Czech word "naprapravit" meaning "to connect" and the Greek word "pathos" for "suffering". This treatment technique for structural imbalances deals with sources of pain which often begin in the spine and spread throughout the body causing locomotor disorders.

Poor posture, trauma from sports injuries or whiplash and even general wear can be the cause of these imbalances which cause the deterioration of the suppleness in connective tissues. Such inelastic tissues produce stiffness which can progress to cause pinched nerves, contributing to health problems like arthritis, carpal tunnel syndrome, Temporomandibular Joint (TMJ) Syndrome and other aches and pains.

The primary method of treatment by Doctors of Naprathy (DN) is manipulation of the spine focusing on the underlying ligaments along with the joints and soft tissues. Practitioners of Naprathy, or Naprapaths, can also use ultrasound, electrical pain relief treatments and heat and cold therapies. To assist treatments they may also use back braces, neckbands, taping and various types of joint supports along with posture and dietary counseling. Patients learn to appreciate their responsibility for their own health with a goal of decreasing dependence on therapy.

The National College of Naprapathic Medicine in Chicago is the oldest and largest school of its kind in the country offering several different programs to receive a DN or Doctor of Naprapathy degree. They are licensed in Illinois and New Mexico, regulated in Ohio and may practice in other states that offer freedom of access statutes.

NATUROPATHY

naturopathic.org or www.anma.com/mon63.html

Naturopathy or naturopathic medicine is a therapy to help the body's ability to heal by employing a variety of techniques. It may use acupuncture, aromatherapy, counseling, hydrotherapy, manual therapy and other techniques. Believing in the healing power of nature, this process recognizes that stressful lifestyles, poor diet and other factors can weaken a person, allowing bacteria and viruses to become a problem in the body.

There are two schools of naturopathy today, naturopathic physicians who may use drugs and minor surgery and naturopaths who adhere to a completely natural and holistic process using the body's natural healing ability. Both treat patients as whole beings with a preference for natural therapies like foods and herbs.

Benedict Lust brought natural health practices like hydrotherapy to America from Germany and opened the first School of Naturopathy in New York in 1905. The concept grew in popularity for a time and then nearly became extinct before gradually being rediscovered by the public in the 1950s.

Today, naturopathic physicians are licensed in 16 states. To become a licensed physician they must have a Doctor of Naturopathic Medicine (N.D. or N.M.D.) or Doctor of Naturopathy degree from an accredited institution and pass the required licensing board exams. Please be aware that a D.N.M. or Doctor of Natural Medicine degree does not qualify to be licensed as a naturopathic physician and carries no regulatory status in this country.

NEW BIOLOGY or Epigenetics
www.brucelipton.com

The science of **epigenetics** is the study of molecular mechanisms used by the environment to control gene activity. This is a paradigm shift about the functioning of the human body, a reversal in the perspective of traditional medicine.

The field is more commonly referred to as the **New Biology** and research scientist Bruce Lipton, Ph.D. is the leading spokesman. His research on cloned stem cells revealed that genes themselves did not control life, but that our biology and behavior are primarily determined by our perceptions of the world, in other words our thoughts, feelings and beliefs. What was once considered magic or metaphysical is today's science.

Cellular and molecular biology research during the last decade is proving to be a catalyst for revolution in conventional medical science. It has shown that cell behavior and genetic expression are directly influenced by information derived from the environment, including energy. Rather than a bottom-up belief where genes within the cell control life, the new top-down philosophy has the nervous system, with its perceptions, attitudes and beliefs, controlling genes. (*also see* **Psychoneuroimmunology**.)

One area demonstrating how thoughts affect human biology is called **neuroplasticity**. With assistance from the Dalai Lama, researchers have begun to discover how years of meditation can change the actual functioning of the brain in an enduring manner.

Dr. Lipton has been a teacher and/or researcher at many outstanding institutions, including The University of Virginia, The University of Wisconsin's School of Medicine, Stanford University's School of Medicine, The University of Puerto Rico's School of Medicine and Penn State University. His ground-breaking book, *The Biology of Belief*, was selected as the Best Science Book in the Best Books 2006 Awards.

OSTEOPATHIC MEDICINE
Website: www.academyofosteopathy.org, www.osteopathic.org

Osteopathic Medicine or Osteopathy is a holistic approach to healthcare recognizing the unity of all body parts and the body's ability to heal itself. A U.S. Army doctor, Andrew Taylor Still, M.D., founded Osteopathy in 1874. In this philosophy of health, a human being is more than simply the sum of its body parts. Osteopathy is considered a separate but equal branch of medical care in this country (having become integrated with mainstream medicine in 1969). However, outside the U.S., where it has remained essentially a drug free system based on manipulative techniques, it is still considered a complementary process.

Doctors of Osteopathy, or D.O.s, receive full medical training of four years of medical school, three to six years of internship or residency and additional training just like mainstream or allopathic physicians. D.O.s receive extra training in the musculoskeletal system, the relationship between the muscles, bones and nerves, so they better understand how a problem in one part of the body can impact other areas.

D.O.s use their hands to help diagnose and treat injury and illness using **osteopathic manipulative treatment** or OMT. This involves moving the muscles and joints with stretching, resistance and the gentle use of pressure to properly align the body. However they also recognize that sometimes medication and surgery may be required therapy.

These are the eight generally accepted principles of osteopathy including concepts like "the body is a unit" and "structure and function are inter-related". They appreciate how body fluids are essential to health and that nerves play a vital role in the motion of fluids. The body can heal itself but maintaining health today is a constant struggle against stress, environmental toxins and other challenges. They believe in a holistic approach to health to prevent illness.

After enduring the horrors of the Civil War battlefield and then the loss of his wife and children from disease, Dr. Still lost his faith in the standard medicine of the day. He began researching and testing other methods of healing and in 1892 founded the American School of Osteopathy in Kirksville, Missouri. His methods attracted a great deal of unpleasant attention at the time and Kirksville was one of the few places that allowed him to practice. Today it's called Andrew Taylor Still University, Kirksville College of Osteopathic Medicine. Although Missouri was willing to grant him a charter for awarding medical doctor degrees, he was so unhappy with the field that he chose to issue his own D.O. degree.

Both Doctors of Osteopathy and Medical Doctors must pass comparable examinations to obtain state licenses to practice medicine and work in fully accredited and licensed healthcare facilities.

PSYCHONEUROIMMUNOLOGY or PNI

www.pnirs.org

Psychoneuroimmunology (PNI) is the specialized field of research that developed from the discovery of neuropeptides in 1972, often called the molecules of emotion. Studying the relationship between behavior, the brain and the body's immune system involves a variety of fields including psychology, immunology, physiology, pharmacology, psychiatry, behavioral medicine and infectious diseases.

Candace Pert discovered this type of receptor while she was still a graduate student. Her 1997 book, *The Molecules of Emotion*, illustrates the challenge of scientific discovery and the difficulty of change in the world of medicine. As neuroscientists have continued to discover more peptide molecules, medical researchers discovered these molecules were also messengers in other parts of the body. This complete, bi-directional circuit is considered scientific evidence of the mind-body connection.

The non-profit PsychoNeuroImmunology Research Society (PNIRS) was incorporated 1993. Its purpose is to promote the study of interrelationships among behavioral, neural, endocrine and immune processes and to encourage collaborations among immunologists, neuroscientists, clinicians, health psychologists and behavioral neuroscientists.

TRADITIONAL CHINESE MEDICINE

qi–journal.com/tcm.asp, www.tcmtreatment.com

The major features of Traditional Chinese Medicine or TCM are herbal medicine, acupuncture and massage, knowledge and techniques which have developed over thousands of years. This medical philosophy believes the functioning of the human body is interconnected and that it interacts with its environment. Diagnosis of disharmony is vital to understanding, treating or preventing illness and disease. TCM is not the same as the original Classical Chinese Medicine (CCM) which was prohibited by the Nationalist government of China for 30 years. TCM is the standardized form of CCM which was developed in the 1960s to focus on its compatibility with modern science.

A large part of the basis of TCM comes from Daoism or the Taoist philosophy. It is believed that the Yellow Emperor composed Basic Questions of Internal Medicine during his reign from 2696 B.C. to 2598 B.C. The first reference to it was toward the end of the second century A.D. Zhang Zhong Jing, considered the Hippocrates of China, mayor of Chang-sha, wrote the *Treatise on Cold Damage* which included mention of the Neijing Suwen.

More information on the elements of TCM can be found later in this work under Acupuncture and Acupressure.

VIBRATIONAL MEDICINE

Vibrational Medicine is a multifaceted concept used to describe a wide variety of techniques to promote the body's natural ability to heal using life-force energy. This may include sound, light, touch, magnetism, homeopathy and many other methods of stimulating an energetic response.

Ancient civilizations across the world developed the original concepts of vibrational medicine with remedies such as flower essences and gemstone elixirs. In time, these formulas and ideas evolved into a fundamental medical system and a form of holistic healing.

The concept is based on the fact that all life is in a constant state of vibrational resonance and harmonics, which produce energy-fields. The healing properties of all any type of vibrational medicine are the result of the unique wave form or harmonics that interacts with the body.

In more modern times, British physician Dr. Edward Bach developed his technique in the 1930s. **Bach Flower Remedies**, or Flower Essences, are made from the flowers' early morning dew and energized by the sun. There are 38 original formulas to correct emotional imbalances by replacing negative emotions with positive ones.

More recently Dr. Richard Gerber's book *Vibrational Medicine* (2001) describes the role of "thought forms" and consciousness in practical terms. The book also explains the benefits of various types of vibrational therapies.

Chapter 2 – Working with the Body

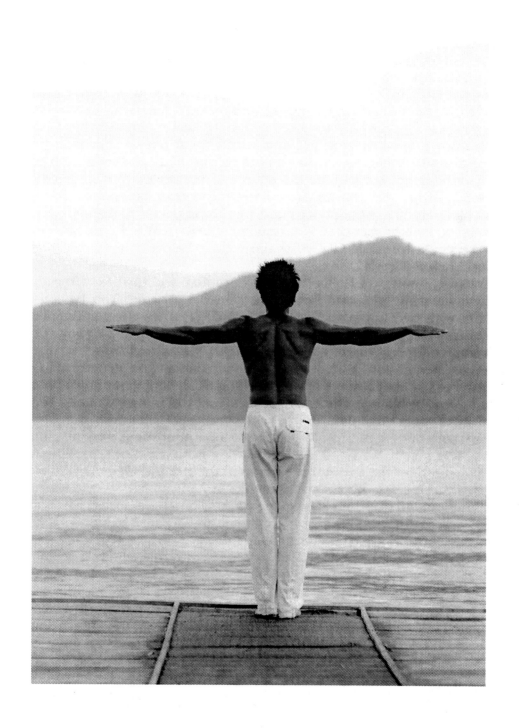

INTRODUCTION TO BODY CATEGORY

Let's begin this exploration into opportunities for health with the body category. In many ways these are some of the easiest subjects to understand because they can be seen and felt. Again, these processes are organized according to my own interpretation of their primary characteristics, you may have a different view. Many are mind-body-energy techniques meaning they could've been placed just as easily in other areas.

The human body is incredible but as you probably already know it can run into trouble. There are a range of therapies in this section which offer ways to restore the body to health, often by finding the real source of the problem. You'll learn about ancient techniques and modern American developments. Some subjects are relatively accepted by the medical community like Dr. Dean Ornish's program while some are still out on the fringe or beyond.

One thing to remember is that a pain or physical problem in one part of your body may not actually be the source of the problem; it may just be a symptom. Let me give you an example from my own experience. For many years I had painful knees and legs and went from doctor to doctor, specialist to specialist, looking for relief. Eventually I ended up at a podiatrist who prescribed expensive custom lifts which did seem to help a little. I wore those lifts for more than a decade.

Last year, I went to a Rolfer for a back problem and the first thing she did was have me walk back and forth. She immediately said "You have a lot of problems with your knees and legs, don't you?" It turned out that the problem wasn't in my feet at all but my whole body. As we grow up and age our body is continually adapting to changes like weight, stress and injuries. In many cases these adaptations ruin our natural body motion and structural integration. After just a few sessions of Rolf work I took the lifts out of my shoes and haven't worn them since. Once my body's structural integration had been repaired there wasn't any pain in my knees and legs.

The happy ending to this story came at the Cotton Bowl football game recently. I was able to walk the mile-and-a-half from the cheap parking to the stadium, stand for the entire three hours of the game and then walk back to the car without any problems or pain. When I got home my wife was absolutely shocked. After all, she'd seen me have so much pain from just walking halfway across our local little shopping mall that I'd have to sit down to rest. This was clearly an incredible improvement!

Using the broken mirror analogy to your health this would represent the physical side of your health, the pieces of broken glass. Perhaps it was a stumble or weakness in your hands that made you drop the mirror. You might have even tried to catch it before it hit the floor and broke but were unable to stop it from its inevitable crash to the floor. As you read these different processes and devices it will be like going backward in time to a point before you lost control of the mirror. You'll discover how to hold the mirror of your health more securely, how to carry it more safely and to treasure it at all times because it reflects your life.

It's interesting that so many of these processes are popular with entertainers since their bodies are strained day after day during performances. Your body may not suffer from similar strains and stresses but it will probably benefit from these techniques as much as professional entertainers and athletes.

A word of warning: you'll find a listing about Nutrition in this section on the Body but there isn't any information about diet or supplements. That's the only subject really not covered in this book, mainly because there are so many different books already available and so many of these therapies have their own nutritional concepts.

To better organize the information in this category it's divided into two basic sections: techniques/processes and devices. As usual the assignment of each subject is completely arbitrary, it's just to make it a little easier to see the similarities and differences in each area.

BODY PROCESSES

ADVANCED JAFFE–MELLOR TECHNIQUE™ (JMT)
www.jmttechnique.com

JMT™ is the abbreviation for Jaffe-Mellor Technique, developed by founders Carolyn Jaffe, Doctor of Acupuncture and Ph.D. candidate in Naturopathy, and Judith Mellor, RN, Ph.D. candidate in Nutrition and certified Chinese medical herbalist. Their combined experience includes various types of acupuncture, herbology and a variety of healing processes.

JMT™ is a bioenergetic therapy that uses **muscle resistance testing** (MRT), a form of applied kinesiology, as the diagnostic tool to identify the pathogenic microorganisms they believe are the cause of many autoimmune diseases. The process may be beneficial for conditions such as osteoarthritis, rheumatoid arthritis, lupus, fibromyalgia, chronic fatigue syndrome, interstitial cystitis, Crohn's disease, colitis, Lyme disease, scleroderma and Multiple Sclerosis. The technique created by Jaffe and Mellor is unique in the way it employs blind testing and focused specific questions to the patient. The original process used vials of materials in the testing process but the process has evolved to the point that vials are no longer used, hence the new designation "advanced".

During the examination, the practitioner views changes in the strength of an isolated muscle against an established baseline. Arm muscles are normally used but any muscle can be used. MRT is valuable as a diagnostic tool because it functions on a subconscious level where the autonomic nervous system resides, the system controlling all bodily functions. In other words ,the process looks around behind the conscious mind to see what's happening inside.

Treatment is a gentle tapping of back muscles with either an activator (a chiropractic adjusting instrument) or an arthrostim, a device that provides mild percussion in rapid succession. The technique elicits the proper sensory input to produce more control of body function by the nervous system. The JMT™ protocol allows for as many as ten corrections during any one visit, but the actual number of corrections varies by condition. Practitioners may dispense homeopathic remedies on a temporary basis to help the body eliminate toxic materials that have built up in the tissues as a result of the disease process.

USER COMMENTS: *"In the summer of 2001...I had nine JMT treatments on my very painful right knee...today I have no pain in the knee and I am able to walk up and down stairs easily and do my favorite work in the garden.*

"I hope many more patients can experience the wonderful relief that JMT offers. Thank you for not only developing this method but also for being willing to train others in the technique."

"Five years ago at the age of 21, I suffered from horrible neck/back pain, migraines, sinus problems, fatigue and joint and muscle stiffness. I felt like my body was decades older than my actual age... During my first treatment, I had mixed feelings because the treatment seemed so very simple. I had to remind myself that the answer is not always a long, drawn out and complex process.

"As the practitioner started to diagnose and name the items I was allergic to, I became more and more convinced that this was for real. The items were completely in line with what my blood test had shown. I also had many environmental and chemical allergies of which I was previously unaware. I was starting to get excited and rightfully so. During the next few treatments, I saw some wonderful things.

"All of my improvements have maintained for months and I am positive that they are permanent. I look forward with great anticipation to what I will experience as my last few allergies are eliminated. I love telling people about JMT at any opportunity and how it has restored my peace of mind, improved my way of life and given me the freedom to make it whatever I want."

ALEXANDER TECHNIQUE (AT)

www.AlexanderTechnique.com

Frederick Matthias Alexander (or F.M. Alexander) developed the **Alexander Technique** to help the body to function more efficiently due to his own medical problems. As an actor who developed chronic laryngitis resulting from his performances he was determined to find a way to heal himself. Eventually he discovered that his problem resulted from excess muscle tension and he realized that if neck tension is reduced then the head no longer presses down on the spine so it is free to lengthen.

The process of how we acquire new movements, constantly adapting and changing from our basic, primary motion can cause health problems. As we grow and continually apply these changes we grow numb to how they differ from our natural motions. Alexander called this principle the Debauchery of the Senses but scientists today label it sensory adaptation. The relationship between the neck and head was the Primary Control and the focal point of his work.

The Alexander Technique applies this principle to improve the freedom of movement for the entire body by reeducation in new ways to sit, lie down, stand up and other daily functions. By teaching the proper amount of energy for an activity the body retains more energy while maintaining greater balance and coordination. The technique is about unlearning the tension the body has accumulated throughout its lifetime and the resulting muscle tension that produces abnormal mannerisms and motions.

The technique is often taught to improve performance in the arts such as music, acting, dance and even in some sports training. The Julliard School of Performing Arts, the Royal College of Music and the Royal College of Dramatic Art in London are just a few of the institutions teaching this technique. It's also used as therapy to aid the recovery of balance and motion, and for speech training to repair the voice. It's even been used to unlearn repetitive stress and to aid those patients dealing with reduced mobility such as those with Parkinson's disease. People of all ages have used the Alexander Technique to improve the quality of their lives for over a century.

Teachers certified by professional societies are often required to complete a 3-year program consisting of more than 1,500 hours of training. Some teachers are trained by an informal, apprentice process. Membership in professional organizations is a matter of personal choice so it is best to learn about any potential Alexander Technique teacher's training prior to beginning any therapy.

USER COMMENTS: *(by permission from website): "The Alexander Technique helped a long-standing back problem and to get a good night's sleep after many years of tossing and turning."—Paul Newman, actor*

"Alexander established not only the beginnings of a far reaching science of the apparently involuntary movements we call reflexes, but a technique of correction and self-control which forms a substantial addition to our very slender resources in personal education." —George Bernard Shaw, playwright.

"I find the Alexander Technique very helpful in my work. Things happen without you trying. They get to be light and relaxed. You must get an Alexander teacher to show it to you." —John Cleese, comedian and actor.

"Mr. Alexander's method lays hold of the individual as a whole, as a self-vitalizing agent. He reconditions and re-educates the reflex mechanisms and brings their habits into normal relation with the functioning of the organism as a whole. I regard this method as thoroughly scientific and educationally sound." —Professor George E. Coghill, Nobel Prize winning anatomist and physiologist.

APPLIED KINESIOLOGY (AK)

www.tfhka.org

Applied Kinesiology (AK) is a technique using muscle testing as a diagnostic tool and for stimulating the body's natural healing ability. Today, there are an estimated 130 variations on this fundamental concept with new adaptations being developed by practitioners frequently. This process is not the same as kinesiology which is the study of movement or physical activity, although many people have confused the terms.

In simple terms, AK uses muscles tests all over the body with no verbal questions and focuses on the structural and nutritional aspects of the body. It also uses gait analysis, range of motion evaluation and other techniques. Many chiropractors, naturopaths, medical doctors, dentists, massage therapists and acupuncturists use the process. Unfortunately, others interested only in selling supplements and some less-than-reputable healing therapies also use muscle testing. Most of the energy or specialized forms of AK use muscle testing as a biofeedback process with only straight-arm (deltoid) muscle tests while asking "yes/no" questions. These practitioners are more concerned about the mental/emotional aspects of the individual.

Although muscle testing had been recognized as far back as the 1920s in the U.S., it wasn't until Dr. Goodheart made his presentation to an American Chiropractic Association meeting in Denver in 1964 that the term "applied kinesiology" became established. His original observation was that a weak muscle could be treated and the strength immediately improved. At first, his work focused on using muscle testing to improve chiropractic adjustments, but sometimes these treatments were not completely successful so he expanded the diagnostic and treatment options.

He noticed specific relationships between muscles and the energy meridians of Chinese medicine. Weak muscle testing would become strong when a patient touched that part of the body where the dysfunction originated, a process he called therapy localization. The process began to use the body's energy system for rapid healing. From these basic concepts, Applied Kinesiology has grown into a broad field of alternative healing.

One of the early pioneers in the field was John F. Thie, a chiropractor in Southern California. When he suggested to Dr. Goodheart in 1965 that his work be made available to the general public, Goodheart told Thie that he should go ahead and do it. He created **Touch For Health**™ (TFH) Kinesiology, publishing *Touch For Health* in 1973 as a self-care approach. Dr. Thie felt the system was so safe and simple that no one needed any training or certification. Today it is one of the most popular types of AK in the world.

TFH muscle testing is a cooperative event involving the practitioner with the active participation by the client. It can be done standing, sitting or lying down and is always done fully clothed. The therapist pulls or pushes against a muscle with about two pounds of pressure for two seconds with a limited range of motion of only two inches or less. If the muscle is weak, "squishy" or simply doesn't lock into place, then the energy within the related meridian is probably not in balance. The therapist can then massage the corresponding points on the body to restore normal energy flow and muscle strength. There are five types of energy systems addressed with the TFH process, but therapists can usually check and balance muscles for all 26 meridians in about 20 minutes.

The International College of Applied Kinesiology (ICAK) was founded in the 1970s and it offers training and certification by its board. Other types of applied kinesiology normally offer their own training and certification programs.

There are many different types of applied kinesiology and this is just a sample. Because different variations use different concepts this subject is categorized for Body, Mind and Energy.

USER COMMENTS: *"I have been suffering from osteoarthritis for a number of years in both knees and my left hip. All the doctor could give me to ease the constant pain was Panadeine Forte which I found to be detrimental to my driving capabilities. I was given 15 minutes of Kinergy treatment and I felt the pain* *leave my body and have had no pain ever since. I also received treatment for my right ankle which used to swell up since being a prisoner of war in 1945. Now there is no sign of the swelling".*

"During a Kinergetics group my system for hair, skin and nails came up as needing work and was dealt with along with other systems. In the following weeks I noticed changes in an indented scar under my eye [it was 40 years old - acquired from a huge boil I got while an underfed student in the 60s]. Within 3 weeks the scar raised up became sore and then completely disappeared. This was an impressive bonus while working on another issue."

"About seven months ago I started sleep-walking, my wife said I should see her kinesiologist since after seeing him she is migraine free after 16 years, so I thought I would give it a try. After the session I told Brett that I had approached four doctors to have them amputate my right leg which was badly damaged in a motorcycle accident 20 years ago. The doctors would not amputate but could not help with the pain. Brett said while I was there would I like to try some Kinergetics pain release on it. I lay back on his table and 15 minutes later I stood up again, the pain had gone from a seven out of ten to a two out of ten. Amazing! I no longer want my leg cut off and I walk four times the distance I could before. Now there is only slight discomfort when I do too much, but is relieved quickly when I rest. It's good to wake up every morning pain free. As for the sleep-walking, I had three session seven months ago and still no sleep-walking. I am amazed that I am pain free after such a long time."

Energy Kinesiology is a term coined by Donna Eden in the 1970s to describe a process of using muscle testing for detecting and correcting imbalances in the body related to stress, nutrition, injuries and even nutritional deficiencies. The Energy Kinesiology Association offers training and certification in its specialty. http://www.energyk.org

USER COMMENTS: *"I told my kinesiologist 'It's just this little issue.' However it took quite a while and another session in the morning but I woke up that Friday (yesterday) and if I stood upright and relaxed my torso would twist. If I really let it relax it would pull my shoulder toward my hip...yes, down. It was amazing to watch. She worked on me with everything she knows and I could track the session by how much twist or discomfort was still there. Inch by inch and pain by pain it all just melted away. Also, on the drive home I got out of the car to go to the rest area and normally I would be stiff from the drive. But I wasn't stiff at all and even more my walk was "loose". Meaning that I felt my hips able to have free motion which I don't think I've had since...I don't know when but I think since about 12 years old when the issue/injury we were working on was started. Because I remember in Junior High thinking I developed my "walk" like other girls do at about that age, but later I realized it was from a dance injury that caused tension in my low back so I would throw one hip forward...I just thought it was the way I walked."*

Health Kinesiology was created by Jimmie Scott as a brand of bioenergetic kinesiology. The process uses muscle testing to identify the priority of the needed work and which energy balancing methods to use. It also identifies the stresses disrupting the energy flow in the individual. For one of his techniques, the Allergy Tap™, he places a substance over a specific acupuncture point on the belly and taps eight pairs of acupuncture points to identify and cure the allergy. http://www.subtlenergy.com/

USER COMMENTS: *"My impression is one of enlightenment. I feel that I have started on the next stage in the journey of my life and have left the baggage of my past behind. It has left me with a thirst for more knowledge about HK.*

I was impressed by the effectiveness of the techniques, their simplicity and the rapidity in getting results. I am particularly interested in the psychological aspect of HK treatment, as it seems to deal straight to the core of the problem however far in the past or subconscious that may be. The results I have seen so far really motivate me into practicing and make me eager to go on further in the study of HK..."

Dawson Program, also known as vibrational kinesiology, was developed by Cameron Dawson. It's based on the concept that the body's emotional, structural, physical and chemical processes are all interrelated so that any change will result in an alteration of the body's energy system. The body contains innate intelligence for constant self-healing and pain and illness are simply a warning system that outside attention is necessary. This process uses muscle testing to locate problems and then applies sound as healing energy. http://www.plusenergi.dk/index.php?id=100

Neuro Emotional Technique® (NET) was developed by Scott Walker, D.C. and is based on the concept that memories are stored in the body which can negatively affect health. NET practitioners use muscle testing to locate a problem event and then perform chiropractic adjustments, use supplements or homeopathic remedies while the client focuses on the problem. See www.netmindbody.com

USER COMMENTS: *I was amazed that a pain in my shoulder could possibly relate to a hassle with a friend in the 3rd. grade and have the pain resolve after NET. That was 15 years ago. Since that time I have been certified in NET and am still amazed how accurate it is and how it shortens my treatment with PTSD clients.*

I developed an extreme posture lean to accommodate my acute back pain. I received an NET treatment and not only did the pain disappear but I immediately stood erect and was able to move about effortlessly.

AROMATHERAPY

www.naha.org

Aromatherapy in the ancient concept of using potent distilled extracts of flowers, fruits, grasses, leaves, spices, roots, woods and other living substances to stimulate the organs, the healing systems of the body and to enhance psychological well being. As a holistic healing process it is able to work on several different levels. Using essential oils the approach delivers various scents to the body directly through the skin by massage or inhaled through the nose.

The use of the olfactory sense provides for an immediate response and easy absorption into the bloodstream. This pathway is especially powerful because it is the only place in the body where the central nervous system is directly exposed to contact with the environment. Once an olfactory cell is activated it sends a signal directly to the limbic part of the brain. In most cases our subconscious mind has already received and reacted to the signal due to our memories and emotions before we're consciously aware of the sensation.

The use of essential oils goes back thousands of years. The Chinese may have been the first to use them along with incense to create harmony and balance. The Egyptians used different types of oils to prepare their dead for entombment and in cosmetics, as medicines and for spiritual purposes. It wasn't until the 16th century that essential oils became available in an apothecary. In 1928, a French chemist by the name of René-Maurice Gatte-fossé created the term aromatherapy as part of his work with essential oils. Today, aromatherapy is growing in popularity as part of the return to more natural types of healing. Properly stored essential oils may last up to 7 years.

The olfactory sense was the subject of the 2004 Nobel Laureate in Physiology or Medicine recognizing that 3% of our genes create olfactory receptor cells which enable human beings to detect 10,000 different odors.

Perfume oils or fragrances are not the same as essential oils since they contain manmade chemicals. However there are synthetic products available which claim to have aromatherapy properties. As with all products, holistic or not, Buyer Beware is a wise precaution.

USER COMMENTS: *"Essential oils are always fun to use because they just smell so nice. They can make you feel better physically as well as emotionally. I haven't tried that many of the different scents but it's amazing how each one produces a different and unique reaction.*

One of the more interesting uses of essential oils is for energy balancing. For example, they can help restore the power of a chakra. Using a pendulum and specific stones to measure the strength of each chakra you can inhale selected essential oils and immediately retest a weak chakra. You'll find it's suddenly strong and vital again as a result of the essential oil.

Aromatherapy isn't just for the holistic crowd anymore. Today even real estate agents are taught to put a pan of water with vanilla on the stove in a model home to stimulate feelings of warmth and a sense of home. Grocery stores make sure the smell of fresh bread or cakes fill the store. Restaurants want to have the aroma of their best dishes filling the air."

ART THERAPY

www.arttherapy.org

Man has always enjoyed and appreciated the healing power of art. The ability to express emotions visually is recognized as an effective catalyst for personal growth and development. Many consider **Art Therapy** a direct development of Anthroposophically Extended Medicine, but it wasn't seen as a separate profession in this country until the 1940s.

Educators have long known that children's artwork demonstrates their emotional and cognitive growth, but psychiatrists began using art created by their patients as part of their healing process early in the last century. The creative process of art can enhance recovery and contribute to health and wellness.

Art therapists are professionals trained in both art and therapy. The regulation of art therapists varies by state so please check the situation in your area when looking for an art therapist. In many areas they can become licensed as counselors or mental health therapists. The American Art Therapy Association was founded in 1969 and is the professional organization for this field while the separate Art Therapy Credentials Board certifies the education and experience of therapists.

ASIAN BODYWORK THERAPY (ABT)

www.aobta.org

Asian Bodywork Therapy (ABT) is based upon Traditional Chinese Medicine although some forms only have roots in TCM. Treatments of the body, spirit and mind with ABT involve restoring the flow and balance of the energy field of life or chi (chee) by manipulation and pressure.

The foundation forms of ABT are *Amma*, *Shiatsu* and *Medical Qigong* but today there are many different forms including: *Acupressure*; *AMMA Therapy®*; *Chi Nei Tsang*; *Five Element Shiatsu*; *Integrative Eclectic Shiatsu*; *Japanese Shiatsu*; *Jin Shin Do® Bodymind Acupressure*; *Macrobiotic Shiatsu*; *Shiatsu Anma Therapy*; *Nuad Bo Rarn*; *Tuina* and *Zen Shiatsu*.

Acupressure – see listing in Energy/Spirit section on p. 121.

Amma – the traditional Korean style of bodywork based upon the Chinese form "Anma". The name means "push-pull" for the style of deep-tissue manipulation used along with acupressure and other points.

Chi Nei Tsang – begins the energy flow in the navel area and then guides the healing power to other parts of the body.

Five Element Shiatsu – relies on the traditional four cornerstones of diagnosis in TCM which are observation, listening, asking and touch. The radial pulse is a key facet of the diagnosis since it often provides crucial information. Locating the disharmony in the body is the basis for determining the best course of treatment.

Integrative Eclectic Shiatsu – combines Japanese Shiatsu with TCM and a Westernized style of soft-tissue manipulation along with dietary and herbal treatments.

Japanese Shiatsu – meaning finger pressure, usually the thumbs, along complete meridian lines.

Jin Shin Do® Bodymind Acupressure – uses deep pressure with techniques to focus the mind and body.

Macrobiotic Shiatsu – is based on the belief that every person is a part of nature. Treatment uses hand and bare foot pressure to improve the flow of chi along with dietary guides, medicinal plants, breathing techniques and corrective exercises.

Shiatsu Anma Therapy – combines the energy system of TCM with modern pressure therapy.

Nuad Bo Rarn – is the traditional Thai bodywork style based upon Indian Buddhist medicine and TCM along with a spiritual focus.

Tuina – is a type of Chinese bodywork using soft-tissue massage along with herbal medicines and therapeutic exercises.

Zen Shiatsu – see listing on p. 70.

The American Organization for Bodywork Therapies of AsiaTM (AOBTA®) is the main professional organization for this field, but the National Certification Commission for Acupuncture and Oriental Medicine (NCCAOM) provides the entry certification for ABT.

USER COMMENTS: *"I was introduced to shiatsu by a friend who was training to become a practitioner. Lucky me! She used me for practice. I had had some "ordinary" massage before, but shiatsu immediately felt special. My learner-friend was methodical and went down the "points" on either side of the spine, and I started feeling my body in new ways. I loved it.*

But that was the end of it until I came to Louisiana and came down with cancer. After my recovery I decided I needed to take better care of myself, and I remembered shiatsu. No two sessions are ever the same with my new practitioner. She takes an inventory beforehand and then magically addresses whatever is ailing me at the time. Magical is a good work for what happens: with astonishingly little pressure, she manages to effect profound changes. I always follow the process with amazement and gratitude, as on a journey, new each time, of discovery of my own body.

I'm convinced, since my cancer these twice-monthly sessions have kept me healthy. If I miss a session I begin to feel it fairly soon. With my intense high-pressure job I crave the release and nurturing of the shiatsu touch and process. It gives me energy and balance and peace. It gives me joy! After every session I wish everyone could have such an experience. The world would be a better, more peaceful place!"

AUDITORY INTERVENTION TECHNIQUE (AIT)
www.BerardAITwebsite.com

Dr. Guy Berard developed an auditory stimulation technique in the 1960s in France following his work with Dr. Alfred Tomatis and the Audio-Psycho-Phonology approach (or Tomatis Method). Practitioners introduced the **Berard Method of Auditory Intervention Training** to the U.S. in 1991 as a method to help people with learning disabilities, autism, ADD and other conditions. Dr. Berard's book, *Hearing Equals Behavior*, was translated into English in 1992.

The premise is that certain people hear differently which impacts their ability to learn and behavior. By using filters to decrease the volume of those frequencies which a person hears too acutely (or peaks) and then randomly modulating frequencies during listening sessions, the AIT sound amplifier can retrain the brain's hearing process. Today Dr. Guy Berard feels the minimum age for this process should be 3 years old.

Practitioners normally take audiograms before, at the mid-point, and at the completion of the sessions to identify and adjust the problem frequencies. The listener will experience 18 to 20 listening sessions of 30 minutes each over a 10- to 20-day period. It's common for people to double up the sessions and have two sessions per day for 10 days. During the listening sessions, the person listens to specially processed music tuned for their hearing situation.

Scientists have found that filtering peaks for the developmentally disabled population is optional since it is the modulation, not the filtering, that is critical for them. The best results normally involve using a multi-disciplinary approach which could include specialists in the fields of audiology, psychology, special education, and speech/language.

USER COMMENTS: (*From a parent about her child):* *"He has changed so much, more than any other year! He gained in social skills, emotional, speech, transitions...His speech therapist has been with him for three years and has never seen him improve as much as he did since AIT. She is truly amazed. He could not write his name before, but within two weeks after AIT he was writing his name. At school he sits in Circle Time; every year before this year he could not sit in Circle Time or any group activity because he said the kids hurt his ears. Now he enjoys all group activities. Now he talks about his friends and he has them over. He used to hate kids touching him, now he just loves his friends. It has been a remarkable year, one of incredible gains for him. Now he is finally ready for kindergarten! Thank you for opening a wonderful new world for our son."*

"I continue to be amazed at the differences AIT has made in my life. I came for AIT in the hope of improving my ability to learn a foreign language. I am pleased to say that everything I had hoped for concerning my ability to learn another language was achieved. My auditory memory/learning ability has also increased. Not only can I repeat longer phrases in French, but I can remember a

phone number when someone says it! Also, my vocabulary is less 'visually de-
pendent'. In a conversation I now 'hear what you mean' instead of only 'seeing
what you mean'.

"Also, I am remarkably more comfortable with other people. To the observer
there was nothing in my behavior that would have revealed my discomfort. In-
deed, others, especially in business, described me as "an extrovert", someone
who was remarkably at ease with others. Not the case. Within, I always felt
"different" than others. I knew that I preferred to be by myself. Social events
that were fun for others were not particularly fun for me. After a few hours of
socializing, I was more than ready to be by myself. Before AIT I had never real-
ized how extremely uncomfortable I had been. After AIT, I came to realize that
social exchanges formerly left me vibrating. I only recognized this when the vi-
brating stopped! I think that I was in a constant "system overload", which I
only recognized once it was gone.

"I wish Berard AIT had been available to me as a child. It would have saved
me from a lot of heartache."

AUTOGENICS TRAINING (AT)

www.autogenic-therapy.org.uk

Autogenics Training (AT) is a self-help technique to generate physical relaxation, bodily health and mental peace. German physician Johannes
Schultz first published the approach in 1932. The term means "self regulation" because it deals with controlling breathing, heart rate, blood pressure
and other body functions. It can also be beneficial in overcoming addictions
such as smoking as well as to change behaviors and to resolve anxieties.

It can take people up to three months to learn and become proficient with
the process. Generally, the training sequence involves a progression of steps
at regular intervals. You can learn and become proficient in the Warm Up
phase in just a few days. However, the first two sequences, often called
Heaviness and Warmth, may require three weeks of practice each. The next
four steps (Calm Heart, Breathing, Stomach and Cool Forehead) each require
two weeks of practice.

While Shultz compared the technique to yoga and meditation, it deals with
the body without any mysticism. It is a method of training the body's autonomic nervous system. Experts believe it functions in a similar manner to
biofeedback, the relaxation response or self-hypnosis.

Autogenics is said to be far more effective than simple Progressive Muscle
Relaxation (PMR) so it's worth the investment of time and effort to learn the
technique. You can also modify the process to deal with specific issues and
problems by inserting visualizations of the negative behavior, its detrimental
effects on your life and then a positive visualization of your life without the
behavior. For maximum effectiveness, it should be practiced on a daily basis.

BIOENERGETIC ANALYSIS

www.bioenergetic-therapy.com

Bioenergetic Analysis or simply **Bioenergetics** is a therapy that uses both the body and the mind to help resolve emotional problems and to help people discover the joy in living. The core principle is the body represents the person - what affects the body affects the mind and the mind affects the body. Muscular patterns in the body, movement and even breathing patterns offer diagnostic tools for the bioenergetic psychotherapist who uses this information to develop a potential framework for the course of therapy. Events in childhood play an especially vital element in the process since they impact adult life and relationships.

Body work as part of the therapy program may take several different forms. For example, Therapeutic Touch is used to facilitate the process. From breathing to handshake to types of movement, each motion of the body offers diagnostic and therapeutic opportunities with this process. Bioenergetics provides increased awareness of the body, the feelings connected to the sensations and to better appreciate how these relate to events in your life.

Dr. Alexander Lowen is the founder of Bioenergetic Analysis. His original work *Bioenergetics* followed his studies with Wilhelm Reich, M.D., an early student of Sigmund Freud, in the early 1940s.

The International Institute for Bioenergetic Analysis was created in 1956 as a membership organization to certify practitioners, provide continuing education and advance the art and science of Bioenergetic Analysis.

USER COMMENTS: *"After years of trying many forms of therapy and medication, I attended a lecture about bioenergetic analysis. My 'inner child' was drawn to the therapist, and my intellect decided this was a modality worth trying. Bioenergetics allowed me to reach places inside that nothing else had reached. Because much of my abandonment issues originated before I had language, the trauma was stored in my body, and no talk therapy could reach it. After much hard work, I finally began liking myself, felt I deserved to be loved and treated with respect, and sensed contact with a Higher Power who wanted the best for me."*

"I have been Rolfed, used Acupuncture, Acupressure, and bioenergetic bodywork which have changed my life. The bioenergetic bodywork deals with both mind and body. I have more energy, think clearly and feel more grounded since I experienced this process. I liked the process so much that I did the training to become a certified bioenergetic therapist."

BIOFEEDBACK

www.aapb.org

Biofeedback is a process of recognizing the functioning of the body's systems in real time with the goal of correcting or improving performance.

Change is accomplished by learning to modify the mind-body connection to alter muscle response, blood pressure and other bodily functions. According to the 2002 federal study on complementary and alternative medicine 1.0% of Americans reported they'd used biofeedback at some time and 0.1% said they'd used it in the previous 12 months.

Many people are familiar with the high-tech equipment often used in movies and sports to improve muscle tone and coordination but a mirror can also be a biofeedback device. When a person simply watches the reflection of each step they're learning to modify the signals from their mind to their body to improve walking. Whether the feedback is done with visual images, sounds or both, it is a process to focus attention to learn improved control.

There are non-invasive devices that will measure muscle tension and brain waves for biofeedback. The term also includes other processes such as:

- **Electromyography (EMG)** – a specialized device used to measure muscle tension, often used as therapy for headaches, morning stiffness and fibromyalgia.
- **Thermal** – the measurement of skin temperature has been found beneficial for Raynaud's Disease and other conditions involving reduced blood flow.
- **GSR** – Galvanic Skin Response is a measurement of the skin's conductivity, usually connected with an audible signal that becomes higher when stressed and lower when relaxed.
- **HRV** - Heart Rate Variability measures changes in heartbeat as a biofeedback tool.
- **Respiration Training** – uses various technologies to train and control respiration.
- **Electroencephalography** or **EEG** biofeedback, also known as **Neurofeedback**, which measures brainwaves by sensors attached to the scalp and each ear. Brain frequency activity is presented so specific frequencies can be stimulated or reduced. The technique has been found beneficial for many problems including ADD, learning difficulties, depression and chronic fatigue.

The technique has a wide variety of uses. It's used by coaches to improve sports performance, by specialists to improve urinary incontinence, to help stroke victims regain functionality and to help people learn to relax, for example. A common feature seems to be dealing with stress. However scientists still cannot explain exactly how biofeedback actually works.

The term started in the late 1960s but certification by the Biofeedback Certification Institute of America began in 1981. There are many state associations which also list biofeedback professionals.

USER COMMENTS: *"My severe tinnitus was making my life miserable. Work was difficult. Reading, thinking, and especially sleeping was a problem. Thanks to Biofeedback therapies I now enjoy life again. Thank you Biofeedback Therapies!"*

"Our grandson has many health issues including ADHD, bipolar, anger and behavior problems and a brain injury from birth. We were told about Biofeed-back Therapies and decided to give it a try. After just a few sessions we noticed a change, he would still get angry but not as long as before. Now he uses the technique he learned when he feels himself getting angry at school or at home and he is able to find the "calm place" that he learned. This has been a miracle for our grandson!"

BIORESONANCE THERAPY (BRT)

www.bioresonance.uk.com/

Bioresonance Therapy (BRT) uses electromagnetic frequencies produced by the body to detect and eliminate health problems. Science knows that all living cells radiate weak electromagnetic energy similar to brain waves. BRT measures this energy to determine healthy and unhealthy conditions along with reactions to specific substances (food, bacteria, and toxins). Practitioners amplify healthy signals and return them to the body to strengthen normal body functions. Unhealthy signals are inverted by a mirror circuit and returned to the body through electronic mats to cancel out the harmful energy. This is the same type of wave cancellation technology used in noise reduction headphones.

The concept for this process is that substances which stress or strain your energetic system are the cause of illness and disease, but it is usually a cumulative effect of several stress factors. Identifying and relieving the major stresses to the system will allow the body to handle the minor ones. Allergy treatments usually take two sessions while infections may take two to four visits. Chronic conditions may require up to eight sessions.

The technology attracted attention in 1991 when Dr. Peter Schumacher used it effectively to neutralize allergies. Study into the concept began in 1923 with the work of Russian scientist Alexander Gurwitsch, but it was German physicist Dr. F.A. Popp who proved the existence of light emission (biophotons) from living cells in 1975. Franz Morell and Erich Rasche introduced Bioresonance Therapy in 1977 with the launch of the MORA-Therapy device. Today there are thousands of BRT machines of many different designs in use around the world by doctors, dentists and even veterinarians to treat a variety of disorders.

The FDA has banned some of these devices from the US market.

BONNIE PRUDDEN MYOTHERAPY®

www.bonnieprudden.com

In 1976, Bonnie Prudden developed her **Myotherapy** method to relax muscle spasms, relieve pain and improve circulation. The technique is based on the concepts of trigger point injection therapy and therapeutic exercise. The term comes from "myo" for muscle and "therapy" for treatment.

"Trigger points" can begin in a muscle whenever it is damaged and are activated by either emotional or physical stress causing the muscle to spasm with pain. The basic formula is:

Trigger Points + Stress + Triggering Mechanism = Chronic Pain.

Older people often suffer from trigger points more as a result of collecting more trigger points.

Myotherapists defuse the pressure by pressing on the appropriate trigger point for several seconds with fingers, knuckles or even elbows and then passively stretching the muscle into its normal relaxed and painless condition. Patients wear loose clothing and no shoes for a myotherapy session. Exercises are taught to each patient necessary for them to remain pain free. Normally patients require less than ten sessions for relief.

Bonnie Prudden's Myotherapy® method is taught in person, through her many books, videos and media appearances. Her work on physical fitness began with her research on the nation's school children in the 1950s which she reported to President Dwight Eisenhower. As a result of her efforts the federal government established the first requirements for children's fitness programs.

Bonnie Prudden Myotherapy is a registered trademark of Bonnie Prudden Myotherapy, Inc.

USER COMMENTS: *"I learned that there is always hope and that I am not stuck in my current condition."*

"I now have reliable information that can easily be incorporated into my work to benefit myself and my clients."

"I call it a recipe book on trigger points and recommend the book (Pain Erasure the Bonnie Prudden Way) to all my patients."

BOWEN THERAPY

www.bowentherapy.com

The Bowen Therapy is a bodywork system that uses cross-fiber muscle movements throughout the body. Tom Bowen created the process in Australia. He was untrained in formal therapy education but had a gift for healing. He began his treatment practice of soft tissue manipulation in the late 1950s and spent his life continually developing his philosophy of healing and his techniques. Unfortunately, he never got around to writing any of it down so today there is some disagreement over his techniques.

The first moves of the Bowen Therapy are done on the back and hips while the client lies face down with only their shoes removed. This initial sequence allows the body to relax, improves the flow of oxygen and circulation while releasing toxins. The series of "moves" in this process are done in a precise sequence across muscle and connective tissues, up and down the body, with the client changing to a face-up position halfway through the treatment. There are short waiting periods during the session which allow the brain to appreciate what's happening and to create a positive response. Sessions usually run 45-60 minutes. The key to the Bowen Therapy is in opening up the body's energy pathways to allow it to heal itself.

Tom Bowen died in 1982 but one of his students, Ossie Rentsch, taught Milton J. Albrecht who was the first Bowen therapist certified outside of Australia. Milton Albrecht sponsored the first Bowen seminar held in the U.S. in 1989. Albrecht founded the Bowen Therapy International organization in 1997 for the competency, certification and quality control of Bowen Therapy practitioners.

USER COMMENTS: *"I was having some shoulder pain and restriction several years ago when I happened to be having breakfast with a good friend who is also a Bowen Therapist. She offered to do some work on my shoulder right in the parking lot of the restaurant. A few simple moves and the pain and discomfort were gone and have never returned."*

"Your Bowen Technique has saved my life! I cancelled my hip surgery scheduled for next week."

"Three visits and the amazing Bowen treatment fixed my frozen shoulder. Thanks!"

BRAIN GYM® or Educational Kinesiology (Edu-K)
www.BrainGym.org

Brain Gym® was developed over a 25-year period by Paul Dennison, Ph.D. and his wife Gail E. Dennison to help children and adults learn more effectively, especially those diagnosed as learning disabled. Beginning in the 1970s practitioners of the process began to use posture and movement to improve academic, interpersonal and physical learning skills. Today, the process uses 26 specific activities that integrate body and mind to produce quick improvements.

They describe the brain as functioning in three dimensions. "Laterality" means the ability of the brain to coordinate both sides of the brain, a fundamental skill to be able to read, write and communicate. "Focus" concerns the coordination of the brain from front to back, critical for comprehension. "Centering" is about the ability of the brain to coordinate the top and bottom areas. This function is vital for organizational skills and the ability to feel and express emotions. Many of the Brain Gym® activities are based on the relationship of movement to perception and their impact on motor and academic skills.

A private session with a trained Brain Gym® instructor or consultant usually lasts 1-2 hours. Each five-step process or "balance" will remove a block and create a bridge in the brain for that specific learning or action goal. The process promotes the ability to learn at a deep, whole-brained level. Short balances may take only five minutes while a longer balance may take an hour or more.

Brain Gym® is a registered trademark of Brain Gym® International / Educational Kinesiology Foundation.

USER COMMENTS: *"Recently, I started to knit a sweater for my granddaughter. The design was an Aran style with cables, diamonds, and bobbles. I soon found myself having dreadful trouble, and had to undo my stitches again and again. So many fruitless attempts! I was ready to give in; no more fancy knitting for me! Then I said to myself, "This is quite ridiculous. I have knitted incredible patterns for years, and I don't believe that you lose this ability just by getting old." As I sat looking at the pattern for the sweater, I thought, "Hang on just a minute, I need to do some Brain Gym." So I stopped and did 20 minutes of Brain Gym activities. No more trouble! The sweater is now finished and much admired, and I've knitted a couple more for my grandson. What's age got to do with it?"*

"We cannot believe the improvement in our daughter after five sessions. Before we were referred to you our daughter could not tie her shoes without help, could not ride her bike without training wheels, and was having difficulty reading at her grade level. Since working with you she is riding her bike without assistance and training wheels. She is tying her shoes by herself, but most important her reading rate and reading fluency have greatly increased, which has also increased her reading comprehension.

We feel that Brain Gym provided the missing link so she could integrate all the previous therapy. Because of your work, she's made huge improvements academically and socially in a very short time period. We are very grateful for your work and thankful that God sent you into our lives."

BREATHWORK

www.rebirthingbreathwork.com/

Breathwork or **conscious breathing** has many different techniques under a variety of names. **Rebirthing**, also called **Rebirthing Breathwork**, is a special breathing technique based on the concept that breathing energy along with air has therapeutic effects on the body. The increase of physical and spiritual energy has a cleansing effect on the body. It is a process to increase awareness of emotions in order to resolve the effects of the past, reconnecting the mind and the body.

Rebirthers don't believe that the past has to be the pattern for the future. It's human nature to suppress those aspects of ourselves that we dislike so we hide feelings of pain, guilt, shame and other negative emotions. Relief is possible using a technique called conscious connected breathing, also known as circular breath, where the client lies on their back or side breathing in and out without a pause. This technique is said to energize the individual with a build up of Chi or life energy. Initially this process is intended for use with a trained and experienced Rebirthing facilitator because this energy could feed negative patterns, which is why Rebirthers provide positive affirmations during the process. Sessions can last one to two hours and many practitioners recommend weekly meetings for at least the first ten sessions.

Many clients do get to re-experience their birth but it isn't the goal of the process. The priority of Rebirthing is to put people in touch with their experience in this moment in time and space, not to offer some type of regression.

Leonard Orr developed Rebirthing in the early 1970s in San Francisco using bathtubs and hot tubs. Eventually the process developed as a dry process to integrate painful experiences from a person's past. He founded Rebirthing Breathwork International, also called Rebirth International, in 1975. Today this organization offers a wide range of training programs.

USER COMMENTS: *"I tried Rebirthing to try and deal with some emotional issues, hoping to find a way to deal with some very traumatic events in my past, especially my childhood. While breathing isn't hard to do, bringing up horrible experiences and feelings right out of a nightmare can be. I went to the sessions week after week and everything just kept getting worse instead of better. I finally quit and discovered a different process which helped me take the sting out of my experiences and build positive, reinforcing new subconscious beliefs about myself and my life."*

Holotropic Breathwork™ was developed by Stanislav Grof, M.D., and Christina Grof in the mid-1970s. Participants breathe deeper and faster than normal for two to three hours, while lying with eyes closed, and listening to evocative music arranged in a specific way. Facilitators, who are certified after extensive training, do not attempt to guide the session; instead participants are encouraged to allow the expression of whatever set of experiences are brought to them by their "inner healers," and facilitators support that expression if needed. http://www.holotropic.com/

CHELATION THERAPY

www.acam.org

Chelation Therapy uses di-sodium **EDTA** to remove mercury, lead, cadmium and other toxic metals from the blood by intravenous infusion, pill or other form. The solution may also be combined with other substances such as vitamins. The process is used for treating atherosclerosis and other health problems following testing of blood, urine or hair to diagnose the need for the treatment.

Decades ago scientists thought that hardened arteries might be softened if the calcium in their walls could be removed, which was the basis for initiating the EDTA treatment. The first indication that EDTA might be beneficial for atherosclerosis came in 1956 when the first reports from doctors announced that patients felt better after treatment. The book *Bypassing Bypass* states that six million chelation treatments have been given safely over the last forty years but it includes warnings of serious side effects.

The 2002 federal study on the use of complementary and alternative medicine in America showed that 0.1% had ever used chelation therapy. The therapy is promoted by the American College for Advancement in Medicine (ACAM).

USER COMMENTS: *EDTA chelation therapy saved my life 2 years ago. I was a hypertensive mess in congestive heart failure taking upwards of 40 Nitroglycerine tablets, as well as high doses of lasix daily just to survive. Since completing therapy I have not used Nitroglycerine in 2 years and only rarely (say 6 months apart) do I use a lasix for excess water retention. This after doctors tried to get me to have Percutaneous Coronary angioplasty with stent placements.*

CHIROPRACTIC
www.amerchiro.org

The principle of **chiropractic** is that energy, especially of the nervous system, must flow freely through the spinal column for good body health. The relationship of the spine's structure and function to the health of the body is a concept that goes back thousands of years to writings in ancient Greece and China. Even Hippocrates, the Greek physician, (of the Hippocratic Oath for doctors) mentioned the importance of the spine to health.

Chiropractors practice a hands-on technique of healthcare. Most people recognize chiropractic care for spinal manipulation or adjustment. Whether an injury is from a single event such as lifting something heavy or from a repetitive stress of poor posture, the result is physical and chemical changes that restrict the movement of the spine. Manipulation, whether manual or by device, restores mobility which reduces pain, muscle tightness and inflammation so the body can heal. Chiropractors often use what's called "passive muscle testing" meaning they observe the lengthening or shortening of the legs or arms in reaction to touching a specific spot to locate the area needing adjustment.

Chiropractic is the largest, most heavily regulated, and best recognized of CAM professions. There are an estimated 60,000 chiropractors in America today. The profession was founded by Daniel David Palmer in Davenport, Iowa in 1895. He began the Palmer School of Chiropractic in 1897 and it continues to be one of the most prominent chiropractic colleges to this day.

Chiropractic care has only recently gained a wide degree of acceptance and respectability. For years the American Medical Association worked to discredit the profession but in 1976 Chester Wilk and four other chiropractors filed a lawsuit for restraint of trade. After 14 years of legal battles a federal court ruled against the AMA, finding that they had engaged in an illegal activity, the use of propaganda against chiropractic.

It requires four or five years of study at an accredited chiropractic college to become a doctor of chiropractic. Each person must also pass national board and all state exams in order to practice. There are also individual state licensing requirements in order to be a chiropractor. Anyone interested in beginning chiropractic treatment should research their state's requirements and the background a potential healthcare professional.

The 2002 federal survey on the use of complementary and alternative medicine in America found that 19.9% had used chiropractic care at some time in their life and 7.5"% had used it in the prior 12 months.

USER COMMENTS: *"If you've ever found yourself on your hands and knees in pain you probably already know how effective chiropractic care can be. Whether it's too much yard work or simply "zigging when you should've zagged" there is nothing like the pain of nerves in the spine!*

"Chiropractors will begin with X-rays and then a careful examination of your entire back. If conditions warrant an adjustment then they'll usually massage the back with a machine to relax the muscles so they'll move more easily. Then they'll hold your feet together to see the length of your legs as a measuring tool for the structure of your spine. It's amazing how they can find each joint that is out of place by your legs, but apparently the stiffness of back muscles changes the relationship of the leg length.

"Adjustments can be made manually in different styles or by the use of a device. The 'Activator' is one of the most common tools to deliver consistent pressure at a precise location. It's not uncommon to get a little of both depending on your situation and needs.

"Today chiropractors are expanding into new technology like spinal decompression tables and even cold lasers to promote spine health. All too often they'll prescribe wellness to keep you out of trouble in the first place."

"I had problems with my legs going numb from my knees down after standing for even a short period of time. After a year with regular adjustments at my chiropractor's office, that has disappeared! Years later, after seeing 3 or 4 different doctors and being misdiagnosed by all, it was my chiropractor who immediately correctly diagnosed my Grave's disease...!"

"I injured my lower back during a cruise to the Caribbean while working out on the rowing machine. The following day it took me well over 30 minutes to move and stand upright after awaking in the morning. I was extremely uncomfortable and experienced lower back pain that made it difficulty for me to seat or to walk. I made an appointment with a friend of mine who is an orthopedic surgeon. Upon examination, he noted that there appeared to be no structural problems but possibly some inflammatory process was responsible for the pain. I was prescribed a muscle relaxant and Valium. After a couple of days of medication, I did not improve with more muscle spasm spreading throughout my lower back and buttocks. I decided to seek a competent Orthopedic Chiropractor and made an appointment for a consultation / evaluation. He took a few X-rays of my lower back and told me that I had a subluxation around my L4, L5 and lower. He also noticed that the muscle spasm had now spread to my upper back. I immediately started adjustments and therapy on the same day. I much say that the first couple of days, I felt more soreness throughout the area. However, each day I began to experience more relief. Slowly, I stared to improve and

was prescribed back exercises to strengthen the areas of involvement. Well, my improvement continued and I most grateful that I did not have to have surgery. My Chiropractor told me that my injury could have resulted in at least two herniated discs since area appeared to be bulging around the L4 and L5. I am most grateful to him for his services since he recognized the problem that was obviously not seen by the Orthopedic Surgeon. Today, I still need to be careful of my back during lifting and exercising but I am free of pain and posses good mobility".

COLONIC HYDROTHERAPY IRRIGATION also Colonic Irrigation or Colonic Hydrotherapy

www.i-act.org

Colonic Hydrotherapy Irrigation, also called a **Colonic** or **Colonic Hydrotherapy**, is similar to an enema. Small amounts of water are frequently mixed with minerals, enzymes or herbs and introduced into the colon using a medically- approved, class II colon hydrotherapy device. Either disposable speculums or gravity-fed systems may be used. The fluid is released from the colon after a short period and the process is repeated several times during the 40-45 minute procedure.

Colonics are often recommended as part of an alternative treatment program to remove toxins from the body which result from processed foods, pesticides and other unhealthy intake. The process has been used since ancient times to treat constipation but current popularity may be due to the late Max Gerson who passed away in 1959. The German physician believed that coffee enemas eliminate poisons and offered a legitimate treatment for cancer. Today colonics and coffee enemas are often used by cancer patients to speed up the removal of radiation and chemotherapy toxins from their bodies.

Caution is advised with this process since there have been cases of medical complications from unsafe or unsanitary practices. Right now it is only regulated in some states; please review the training and certification of your practitioner along with your state requirements. The International Association of Colon HydroTherapy offers standards and certification.

USER COMMENTS: *"When I was an Air Force pilot doing high-altitude work I trained my body not to defecate so I could fly the 12-hour missions without having to go to the bathroom. At that time I was only having bowel movements every three or four days, sometimes once a week. My doctor said that's just the way it is and prescribed laxatives.*

Once I retired I discovered colonic hydrotherapy and it's been incredible to get my body functioning again normally. It's a great feeling to be able to go to the bathroom regularly!"

CRANIOSACRAL THERAPY (CST) also Craniopathy and Cranial Osteopathy

www.craniosacraltherapy.org

Craniosacral Therapy or CST is based on the belief that all living tissues have a motion of life which produces rhythmic impulses. This "Breath of Life" was discovered by osteopath Dr. William Sutherland more than 100 years ago. He realized that cranial bones were designed to provide a small amount of motion which he compared to the motion of gills on a fish. These movements involve a network of tissues and fluids at the core of the human body such as spinal fluid, fluid surrounding the brain and the central nervous system. The ability of cells and tissues to express this primary motion is a vital feature for determining our general health.

Manipulation of the skull has been practices for thousands of years, going back to Egypt, India and even Peru. Dr. Sutherland began to teach his therapeutic techniques to remove restrictions in this motion to other osteopaths in the 1930s. Dr. John Upledger began teaching what he called "craniosacral therapy" in the mid-1970s to people not trained as osteopaths.

There are at least three different rhythms in this "primary respiratory system", each with its own rate of vibration and pulse. These pulses are identified as: the cranial rhythmic impulse; the mid-tide and the long tide. CST practitioners listen through their hands to the patient's body rhythms to detect any patterns of congestion or restriction. They then apply gentle pressure to improve the functioning of the central nervous system so the body can better heal itself.

There is also a type of massage called Craniosacral so it's best to check the training and qualifications of your therapist, it could be simply a head massage instead of therapy.

The Craniosacral Therapy Association of North America was founded in 1998 to promote the therapy, offer recognition and registration for Craniosacral Therapists. In the U.S. the process has a variety of licensing requirements so check your local regulations.

USER COMMENTS: *"This feels amazing when it's done right, like your brain is being centered. I feel my sinuses start working again and there is a sense of relaxation that flows through my entire body. It literally feels like your body is unwinding from all of the tension. It also leaves you with a sense of wholeness, like you're back to square one being yourself again. Good stuff but I've found a wide range of techniques. Some therapists really know what they're doing and some are just doing a gentle scalp massage".*

"I experienced this as a very gentle subtle form of healing. The practitioner did touch me but the touch was very light. My legs were gently manipulated. There were times when I was asked to tune into my body and give feedback about what I was experiencing. It was deeply relaxing. I felt as though I was floating."

DIGESTIVE HEALTH THERAPY

www.americanherbalistsguild.com,   www.enzy.com/digestion/

There are several different facets of **Digestive Health Therapy**. First there is the general health of the five parts of the digestive tract and its estimated 10,000 different organisms. The small intestine is 15 to 20 feet long and that's where most digestion and absorption of food takes place. Food has always been medicine (remember chicken soup?) and herbal medicine today offers unique advantages for treatment of the digestive system. While there are almost as many self-help books as there are supplements today, the services of a skilled herbalist may be beneficial in diagnosing individual dietary requirements.

There are also specialized fields of Digestive Health Therapy. **Enzymes** or **Enzymatic Therapy** are the biggest area because they're required for almost all chemical activity in the body from digestion, to building bones, for repairing tissues, purifying blood and aiding in detoxification. They are reported to be beneficial for many degenerative diseases by reducing inflammation. Enzymes are reduced in our food today due to processing so the addition of natural food enzymes, corrective dietary habits and whole food supplements in the diet can improve health by improving the digestive system.

Pioneering research into the importance of enzymes goes back more than 50 years with the work of biochemist Dr. Edward Howell. Today we know there are different types of enzymes: dietary; digestive; systemic and metabolic. Dietary enzymes are found in all natural unprocessed foods and aid in the digestion and breakdown of that food. Digestive enzymes are produced by the pancreas and secreted into the stomach and small intestines to aid food enzymes in the digestive process by pre-digesting foods. Metabolic enzymes are produced by the liver and control most chemical reactions in the cells. Systemic enzymes act as catalysts to start and stop chemical reactions such as immune function and hormone balance. Unlike other enzymes these must pass through the stomach to be released into the blood stream.

USER COMMENTS: *"Most people don't realize that those self-help products you find at the health food store can also do a great deal of harm. I took a product to cleanse Candida out of my digestive system (being so very well self-diagnosed) and it worked great the first time. I had no symptoms for a year and felt the best I had in ages. However when I tried the same product again the entire digestive tract went haywire. Nothing I've tried worked and eventually I ended up at the Mayo Clinic."*

"It's taken a lot of time to rebuild the enzymes and thousands of chemical reactions in my digestive system. The natural balance of this entire flora isn't known to current science and it is such a complicated system you really need to proceed with caution and care. Even when under the supervision of a medical doctor or herbalist exercise extreme caution because you'll be the one to suffer through the trial-and-error of correcting your digestive tract!"

DOULA

www.dona.org

Doula means the continuous emotional and physical support for women during labor and early postpartum so they can experience satisfying childbirth and postpartum events. The term "doula" describes a woman serving other women. Dr. Marshall Klaus noticed in 1967 that many parents of premature babies were having difficulty adjusting, partly because standard medical practice at that time was not to allow mothers into the premature nursery until immediately before discharge. Dr. John Kennell joined with Dr. Klaus to study bonding and their work was instrumental to opening nurseries to parents and to allow parents of normal, full-term babies to be with infants during the first moments after birth.

In the late 1980s and early 1990s, researchers found that women who had used doulas had shorter labors and fewer caesarean births. Recent research shows women who have doula support also have increased rates of breastfeeding, more positive mother-infant relationships and greater satisfaction with their birth experience.

Doulas support families emotionally to help them feel comfortable with the experience. DONA® International was started in 1992 by Drs. Klaus, Kennel along with Phyllis Klaus C.S.W., M.F.C.C., Penny Simkin PT and Annie Kennedy to promote doula care. Today there are nearly 6,000 members worldwide. The association provides training and certification.

USER COMMENTS: *"My doula was indispensable. She helped me move from position to the other, whispered encouragement in my ear, taught me how to moan lowly and loved me in a time of great need. This resulted in a safe, and quick, natural birth with no drugs and no interventions.*

"She acted as an advocate for me. Physically, when I was ready to push, I was shaking badly. She knew little tricks of rubbing my toes that would keep my jaw from chattering. She took photographs, so we didn't have to worry about that. When I finally asked for the epidural, I was nervous about it, but she supported me and did not make me feel guilty at all for getting pain relief. It was just very reassuring to have someone with so much knowledge there, and to have a kind and warm spirit to help us through the whole experience.

EAR CANDLING

www.thermo–auricular.com, www.earcandling.com/,
en.wikipedia.org/wiki/Ear_candling

Ear candling is a simple, safe way of removing excess wax and toxins from inside the ears. The process has been used for thousands of years in Egypt, Tibet, India, China, by American Indians and European healers. Today it's used by Amish, in Europe and by others interested in natural healing techniques. It's also called Thermo-Auricular Therapy and Ear Coning.

Originally the straws used in the process were made of pottery clay carved to create a downward spiral of heated air which would carry the smoke of herbs into the ear. The flow also creates a vacuum inside the cone to draw out excess waste and impurities. Today a wide straw of unbleached cotton cloth coated in wax or other material is used to create vacuum to draw excess ear wax and toxins into the straw in a 30-45 minute process.

The procedure is done with the client lying on their side with a towel wrapped around the ear. The practitioner gently places the narrow end of the cone into the entrance of the ear canal. A paper plate or other collection device placed at the middle of the candle to collect the melting wax. When the candle is lit the convection process draws the warmed and softened ear waxes up and into the straw bringing out any impurities, toxins or allergens. As the candle burns it's normal to hear crackling and hissing. Many people report the warmth provides a soothing and relaxing experience.

There are many different types of ear candles. Some are made with different types of oils or herbs in the wax for different effects. For example, Biosun candles are very popular in Europe because they do not have any chemical pesticide & fungicidal residues and carry the prestigious CE mark (93/42-EEC class 11a) for medical devices in Europe. Food and Drug Administration regulations prohibit ear candles from being sold or advertised in America as medical devices.

There is a wide range of training for practitioners; some simply have started practicing after being patients. CAUTION is advised since there have been reports of burns and damage to ears from inexperienced therapists and improper use of materials. Also do not use this process if you have a punctured ear drum or other injury to the ear.

USER COMMENTS: *"My daughter and I do ear candling on each other because it's so easy. It's a warm and delightful feeling and it does wonders for my sinus headaches and allergies."*

"I had been having vertigo for two months; the day after the ear candling session, it was gone. I had a directional hearing problem in my left ear that was also alleviated after the session."

"I've had problems with my ears since my youth. I remember having several ear infections as a boy and as I grew up, I noticed moderate changes and discomfort in my ears throughout my adult life. The ear candling session immediately alleviated the wax build-up. Right away there was a noticeable improvement in my hearing."

EMEI QIGONG

emeiqigong.com

Emei Qigong is also known as Er mei Qi Gong and Er Mei Chi Gong is an extensive system of which therapeutic practices are but one small part. The Emei Qigong medical system includes Energy Transmission Healing Methods, the Energy Information Healing System, and the Emei Qigong Therapy External Energy Diagnosis and Treatment System. This form of Qigong was created in 1227 by a former Taoist priest who became a Buddhist and is based on the heart of the Mahayana/Vadrayana tradition of Buddhism. Emei Qigong is also sometimes known as the Emei Sudden Enlightenment School.

Emei Qigong is based on the understanding that Qi, or vital energy, is a unique form of matter that can be heard, seen, felt, and transmitted through spiritual channels. It also stresses the cultivation of heart to increase virtue and eventually reach enlightenment. The three facets of the methodology are motion and movement, quiet and meditation, and a combination of motion and meditation.

Emei Qigong practitioners treat the human body holistically and view the universe and the human body as a combined and integrated system. They understand that we become sick when we have exhausted our energy, and that we can treat physical, emotional, and spiritual diseases by balancing and replenishing the internal Qi (life force energy) with universal energy. Proper breathing and a balanced mental state are vital to correctly practicing Qigong forms, they're also considered the basis for good health. Using Emei Qigong techniques it's possible to generate good health to a level where you're supposed to be immune to diseases.

Emei Qigong has its own medical system that has been passed down from ancient times and while it differs in many respects from Traditional Chinese Medicine there are also similarities. The Emei Qigong therapeutic system includes acupuncture, acupressure, tuina, moxibustion, herbal therapies, diagnosis, and more so it forms a complete medical system.

The late Abbot of Guang Ji Temple in China, His Holiness Ju Zan, who was the 12th Lineage Holder of Emei Qigong as well as the Supreme Abbot of Chinese Buddhism, empowered Grandmaster Fu Wei Zhong with the mind/heart transmission of the Emei Sudden Enlightenment School after Fu had studied with him for eight years. Grandmaster Fu is the 13th Lineage Holder, a position that goes back 800 years.

Grandmaster Fu feels that the essence of Qigong is more than creating vital energy. He teaches that cultivating virtue and attaining enlightenment bring true happiness and empowerment into our lives. He left China in 1995 to bring Qigong to the United States and other Western countries. Because of cultural differences between the East and West, Grandmaster Fu devoted himself to adjusting his teachings to make them accessible to Western people. He has developed a structured course of study that is systematic, practical, easy to learn, and quickly effective. Currently, he teaches four levels; as students become ready, he will add higher levels.

Level One, the first course, teaches all of the basic theory as well as techniques to heal the self as well as others. Level Two training is called "Change the Moving Program of Life" and teaches students how to find their balancing element based on their four pillars. It also teaches a special meditation that will balance students' pre-birth energy and improve their karma. Level Three is called "Yi Jing and Heart Energy Distinctive Healing Methods." At this level, students learn how to find the root causes of chronic diseases, including cancer, heart disease, auto-immune disorders, and so on. They also learn how to heal these diseases after finding the root cause. Level Four is called "Emei Qigong Level One Teacher Training." As Emei Qigong Level One teachers, students must be able to teach, heal, and organize official seminars. Emei Qigong's healing processes and heart-based, virtue-building practices can make a great contribution to caring for physical, emotional, mental, and spiritual health.

Currently, Grandmaster Fu spends most of the year in China, training the monk who will share the position of 13th Lineage Holder. The monk Lineage Holder's responsibility is to preserve the purity of Emei Qigong and pass it down to the succeeding layman Lineage Holder. Grandmaster Fu also spends a few months a year in North America, training future Emei Qigong teachers in the hope that one day, when he retires, Emei Qigong will be able to continue on, in its purity, in the West.

USER COMMENTS: *"In 2000, I was introduced to Emei Qigong. My friends, family members and I were in awe of the changes I experienced once I became interested and involved. Prior to practicing and cultivating Emei Qigong, I can admit to having been very overweight, depressed, lethargic and generally speaking, I was obsessively preoccupied with how out of control my life was and how hopeless I felt. My past behavior can be best described as over-reactive, defensive and very angry. T.V. Judge Judy's team wanted me on their show after reading a 1999 police report filed due to an unfortunate incident with my now "wasband." I have been able to resolve my challenges and restore my faith in myself and mankind by being a dedicated student and by practicing all the Emei Qigong techniques offered. I now enjoy being more balanced emotionally, physically, psychologically, and spiritually. I am kinder to myself and others and can enthusiastically share with others the benefits one can experience from practicing and cultivating this amazing Art and Science."*

"I have been an Emei Qigong practitioner for six years now and I can speak from personal experience about the difference that this type of energy healing has made in my life. At first when I finished my level one training, I went home and started practicing Wuji Gong with the video from Grandmaster Fu.

"After a couple of weeks I began to notice a significant change in my health and I also noticed that I walked differently; meaning I had a more fluid gate when I walked, and I thought this was nice I was moving very gently through my path. The next thing I noticed was that my back pain had disappeared and that my blood pressure had stabilized. As I continued training with Grandmaster Fu, I learned how to do healing on others as well as myself."

FELDENKRAIS METHOD®

www.feldenkrais.com, www.feldenkrais-method.org

The **Feldenkrais Method**® is a process of educating the body which expands the assortment of movements, enhances awareness, improves function and enables people to express themselves more fully. It is very popular with dancers, musicians and artists. It can be used by anyone who wants to reconnect with their natural ability to move, think and feel. It is also effective at improving movement-related pain and functioning in cases of stroke or cerebral palsy. It is not a massage, bodywork, or necessarily a therapeutic technique, it's a learning process.

A core belief of the Feldenkrais Method® is that improving the ability to move can improve one's overall well being. It is based on principles of physics, biomechanics and an empirical understanding of learning and human development. The Method is an educational system that uses movement and awareness as the primary method for learning and its purpose is to give greater functional awareness, defined as the interaction of the person with the outside world or the self with the environment. By teaching people how their whole body cooperates in any movement helps them live their lives more fully, efficiently and comfortably.

The Feldenkrais Method® is expressed in two parallel forms. **Awareness Through Movement**® lessons are organized around a particular function and normally last 30 – 60 minutes. There are hundreds of hours of these verbally-directed movement sequences which evolve from comfortable, easy movements into movements of greater range and complexity. **Functional Integration**® is a hands-on form of tactile, kinesthetic communication. The practitioner communicates to the student how they organize their body by gentle touching and movement which shows how to move in more expanded and functional ways. The lesson is usually performed lying on a table designed specifically for the work but it can also be done with the student in sitting or standing positions.

Moshe Pinhas Feldenkrais moved to Tel Aviv in 1954 and made his living for the first time solely by teaching his Functional Integration method. In the late 1950s Feldenkrais presented his work in Europe and The United States. In the mid-1960s he published *Mind and Body* and *Bodily Expression*. In 1967, he published *Improving the Ability to Perform*, titled *Awareness through Movement* in its 1972 English language edition.

The Feldenkrais Guild® of North America provides accredited Training Programs which are required to be certified, to become members of FGNA, and to use its service marked terms for The Method. Feldenkrais®, Feldenkrais Method®, Awareness Through Movement® and Functional Integration® are registered service marks of the Feldenkrais Guild® of North America.

USER COMMENTS: *"The Method creates a smoothness of motion that is absolutely wonderful. The motions can be so small and subtle that you don't feel a thing, until the next day. Then you can be sore as hell! It's amazing how* *such miniscule changes in posture or motion can have such big repercussions in your whole body."*

"Feldenkrais is a lot less invasive than Rolfing and it's focused more on connecting the mind to the body so the muscles move the way they're supposed to, it's a much more subtle process. After a session I usually walk a couple of blocks just to rediscover my body and it's amazing how much lighter it feels and how much more fluid my movements are."

"As an aging ex-jock, nursing bad knees and shoulders, Functional Integration® and Awareness Through Movement® work helps me develop insight into how my body operates and how it compensates for old injuries. With a more solid understanding of 'what is,' I can start to make intelligent choices about how I want to move, sit, stand and just function."

FLOATATION THERAPY
www.floatationfederation.com, www.samadhitank.com/

Floatation Therapy, originally known as sensory deprivation, was created in 1954 by Dr. John C. Lilly, an American neurophysiologist and psychoanalyst. He expected to learn about the brain in sleep states but discovered that the mind becomes more even more active when deprived of outside stimulation. It's also been called **Restricted Environmental Stimulation Technique** (REST) since the 1970s. The process produces profound relaxation which allows the mind and body to regenerate natural energy without interference. There are similarities between this process and some forms of meditation.

There are two major types of floatation devices, wet or dry. Clients float directly in the water in the wet version, but rest on a sheet of plastic on top of the water in the dry version. Most floatation tanks measure about eight feet long and four feet wide and contain just enough very warm water to float. The water has loaded with salts and minerals making it nearly impossible to sink. Clients will shower before and after each session which may last from one to two hours. There are variations depending on customer preferences such as complete darkness or having a little light and having the tank completely closed or having the lid left open slightly. Some people prefer total quiet while others request soft music or even self-hypnosis tapes for losing weight or to stop smoking. There is usually a 2-way microphone built into the tank for communication.

The deep relaxation produced by this environment has beneficial effects on the body, primarily in increased healing capacity. There are also psychological benefits connected with the process. By reducing stress it's been useful in the treatment of obsessive and addictive behaviors. Floatation tanks may be found in health clubs and spas or purchased for home use.

There are warnings about this type of therapy is you have a history of psychological disorders, especially claustrophobia.

USER COMMENTS: *"This is how I feel about floating: I am light and expanded within a safe cocoon of space. It is filling, simple and complete. Mainly I know I'm doing something very good for me. It is a healing, an acknowledgement, a growing. It is a good thing."*

"So, there I was in darkness and silence, floating. It was as black as black could be, silent as a tomb. The water was so buoyant that I floated right on the surface, feeling as secure as I would on a rubber mattress and a lot more comfortable. I soon felt more relaxed than I ever had in my life, free of gravity, floating in warm, silent peaceful space, alone with my mind. Then I realized that I no longer had a body, but the discovery didn't upset me, I didn't even bother to wiggle my fingers—the perfect repose of floating, the stillness of silence was too sublime, too euphoric to disturb. And it occurred to me that all sorts of interesting, exciting things were happening in this black, empty nothingness."

HELLERWORK STRUCTURAL INTEGRATION
www.hellerwork.com/

Hellerwork Structural Integration combines deep-tissue structural bodywork, movement education and dialogue to restore the body's natural balance. It's based on the concept that the body, mind and spirit are inseparable so they must be treated as a whole.

Therapy is customized to each individual but built on a standard 11-step series. Most of the work done in the one-hour sessions takes place on a massage table but sitting or standing work may also be included. The process first works with the connective tissue to realign the muscle-skeleton system to restore balance and ease of motion. Movement education trains the person to move with minimum effort. The dialogue process explores how thoughts, beliefs and attitudes impact the body. Hellerwork feels like slow deep pressure that is followed by a sensation of release. Clients may need to make slow motions while the practitioner guides the tissue. Practitioners are trained in the amount of pressure to use, speed and technique but sensations may vary from pleasure to mild, temporary discomfort based on the condition of the tissue.

Hellerwork believes that everyone is innately healthy but to maximize your health you must develop deeper experience with your movement, the integrity of your body and your relationship with yourself and your world.

Joseph Heller was born in Poland in 1940 but came to the U.S. at age 16. He studied with Ida Rolf, the originator of structural integration, becoming a Rolfer in 1972. He also studied Structural Patterning from Judith Ashton. He became the first president of the Rolf Institute in 1975 and continued studying with Ida Rolf until 1978 when he left the Institute to create a new type of bodywork called Hellerwork.

Training and certification is done by Hellerwork International. As a type of bodywork it requires massage licensing in most states. Please check the training, qualifications and licensing of your practitioner before beginning any type of bodywork therapy.

USER COMMENTS: *"Hellerwork has been the least amount of effort, the least amount of time, the least amount of money for the greatest amount of benefit of anything I have ever done."*

"I was a professional hockey player for 20 years ... (after) Hellerwork ... my posture was better, joints moved easier, I could breathe easier and this was only after a few sessions."

"As an old nurse, my back has taken me on a magical mystery tour of alternative health ... Hellerwork helped me the most, not just in simple symptom relief (though there is no finer bodywork system) but in the process of developing a relationship with my poor, abused and ignored body. Since completing the series ... I have enjoyed happy good health, and a two way communication with my lumbar spine, which in a friendly way reminds me when I need to pay it more attention."

HERBAL BODY WRAP

Herbal Body Wraps were created to shrink the size of the body, offering a slimmer body very quickly. There are a wide variety of products and treatments available using an assortment of ingredients. There are self-help products to use at home and treatments available at spas or from your local massage therapist.

Body Wraps claim to work by shrinking fat cells by assisting them to release toxins, firming and toning the skin. Others claim that success lies in its ability to compact the body. Clay wraps are said to function as a poultice to draw impurities from the body. Skeptics say it simply dehydrates the body so any size reduction is temporary and will be lost as soon as the body is hydrated with fluids again.

The process may use a proprietary blend of herbs and minerals, sea vegetation, sea salt, sea mud, aloe vera, amino acids and other ingredients. Cloth strips are soaked in the solution and wrapped around portions of the body or the entire body which makes you look like an Egyptian mummy. If only portions of the body are wrapped then trapped wastes may simply move from one part of the body to another instead of being eliminated. When you're properly wrapped in cloth strips you are then wrapped in plastic or wear a rubberized outfit to retain body heat, and simply lie in your tub at home or on a table at the spa for about an hour.

In general, licensed massage therapists can do body wraps for muscle relaxation and rehabilitation in most states and estheticians can do body wraps for the purpose of beautifying the skin. Regulations vary so please check with your appropriate state licensing agency. There are also a variety of products designed for home us available in stores and on the Internet.

USER COMMENTS: *"Thank you for The Body Wrap! In just one month I am 36" smaller, my body looks and feels great! My skin is much smoother and I have much more energy. Keep up the good work!"*

"When I first discovered The Body Wrap about 3 years ago, I had lost some weight - from 200 lbs. down to 179. Also, over this period my weight was down to 130 lbs. and never during the weight loss did my skin appear baggy or loose. I was very pleased with the smooth, toned appearance of my skin. I am very pleased with the results I have experienced and look forward to my wraps."

HYDROTHERAPY or Hydropathy
http://en.wikipedia.org/wiki/Hydrotherapy

Hydrotherapy is using water for health and **hydrothermal therapy** adds temperature, as in hot baths or saunas. This is one of the oldest forms of therapy going back to ancient Greeks. Public communal baths were also part of ancient Rome. China and Japan also had bathing as part of their ancient cultures. Being immersed or doing exercises in water has been a popular therapy in many cultures for thousands of years.

There are many different methods of hydrotherapy including: baths and showers; **colonics**; douches; localized therapies like sitz or foot baths; steam inhalation; hot compresses and body wraps to name just a few. The healing properties of water are based on its mechanical effects (either pressure or jets) or its thermal effects. In addition various herbs or salts may be used to enhance the experience. Heated water in a whirlpool or bath naturally soothes the body while the weightlessness of being in water helps to relieve stress. When pressurized jets are used circulation is boosted helping to release tight muscles. From spas in Europe to thermal springs across America like Hot Springs, Arkansas and Palm Springs, California, hot water therapy has always been popular. These naturally heated hot springs often contain a variety of minerals which are promoted as having special healing powers.

A **sauna**, also called a Turkish or hot air bath, can have temperatures of 120 to 212 degrees with 150 degrees Fahrenheit being the norm. There are also moist air steam baths. In either case, the heat stimulates the body to sweat toxins out through the skin. They also stimulate blood flow, increase heart rate, open airways and promote hormone production. Exposure can range from twenty minutes up to two hours. This is similar to the sweat lodge used by American Indian tribes.

Another common type of hydrotherapy is a wrap, either hot or cold. Primarily used as a supportive measure for treating fever and local inflammation, a moistened cloth is wrapped around the body or its affected part and then covered with a dry cloth. If a cool wrap is used to reduce inflammation the process will probably last 45 minutes to an hour. If a warm cloth is used to produce sweating the procedure may last hours.

When using a spa or hot tub a neutral temperature ranging between 92 and 94 degrees is recommended to relieve tension but a higher temperature of 102 to 106 degrees is often suggested if the goal is to relax muscles. Taking a cold shower after a hot bath can be very invigorating!

Please consult your doctor to determine if this type of therapy is suitable for your condition. Many people should avoid this type of therapy. People with diabetes should avoid any hot body wrap but especially to their feet or legs. Immersion in hot baths or using hot saunas is not recommended for diabetics, pregnant women, and people with multiple sclerosis or anyone with abnormally high or low blood pressure. The elderly and children should also exercise caution. Always be sure to drink plenty of water to replace what's been lost!

USER COMMENTS: *"A hot tub is fine and my personal Jacuzzi tub is wonderful after a strenuous day but there is nothing like the full treatment at a spa. One of the main reasons for visiting Hot Springs, Arkansas was to enjoy a real hot spring dip and massage. The water is heated deep in the earth and comes up at 147 degrees so it's mixed with cooler water for comfort. There are ancient American Indian legends about the healing powers of the Valley of the Vapors so in 1832 Congress created the first federally protected area in the national park system for these thermal springs.*

There are plenty of choices along Bathhouse Row but we chose the historic Park Hotel which was opened in 1930. The history seemed to ooze out the walls, from Prohibition to visits by President Franklin Roosevelt to modern times. You have your choice of just how hot you want your own hot spring bath. The massage afterwards was too short and basic but incredibly relaxing. There are even faucets in the park and along Bathhouse Row so anyone can fill up a jug of this special water to drink. We took home several bottles."

LYPOSSAGE™

www.lypossage.net

Lypossage™ was created by Charles W. Wiltsie III, a licensed massage therapist in Connecticut, to help women lose size without losing weight and help them reduce the appearance of cellulite. He came up with the original idea in 1998 and today Lypossage™ has become part of both the massage therapy and the health and spa industries.

Lypossage™ can be done manually or with the G5 Lypossage™ 3 Zone Massage Machine to improve appearance without liposuction, or to complement cosmetic surgery. Stalled lymphatic fluid can cause unsightly and unwanted bulges so Lypossage™ helps to cleanse the body, improve lymph flow and break up the connective fibers that hold fat in the dimpled areas. It also helps to tone muscles and firm sagging tissues, especially in the lower face and neck area along with the buttocks and upper thighs.

Only professionals trained by Pro-Actif Spa Systems International, its certified Master Trainers or 5 Star Educators may use the trademarked term

"Lypossage™". To find an authorized Lypossage professional visit their website listed above.

USER COMMENTS: *"As your slogan says, I now feel as good as I look. I have energy now and enjoy spending more time playing with my kids. I now can get a full night's rest without waking up every hour. Best decision that I have made to help improve myself."*

"I tried everything under the moon to fit into my favorite dress and by the time I completed the Lypossage™ Treatment, the dress was too big!"

"By age 45, my waistline was almost nonexistent. After just three sessions of Lypossage, I've lost over an inch from hips and waist. More important is an increased energy level and the ability to move my body like I could at age 25! I can't wait to do all 18 sessions."

MANUAL LYMPHATIC DRAINAGE (MLD) also Lymph Drainage Therapy (LDT)

www.vodderschool.com, or

www.garynull.com/Documents/Arthritis/Lymph_Drainage_Therapy.htm

Manual Lymphatic Drainage was created in the early 1930s by Danish scientist Dr. Emil Vodder as a series of massaging motions for the relief of chronic sinus congestion and immune disorders. Later it became a major therapy for the management of Lymphedema, a swelling in the arms and legs caused by the accumulation of lymphatic fluid.

The majority of the lymphatic system is located just below the surface of the skin using body motion to move fluids to the kidneys and liver for elimination. Injury, infection or surgery that removes the lymph nodes can slow or block this flow of fluid resulting in Lymphedema.

MLD uses a range of specialized and rhythmic motions to stimulate the lymphatic vessels. Light sweeping movements promote the flow of lymph into the capillaries near the surface of the skin. Stronger motions push the lymph to flow more deeply into the tissues. There are also specialized MLD movements to soften problem tissues. There are several major styles of this therapy including the Vodder, Foldi, and Leduc or Casley-Smith. Sessions normally last 30 to 60 minutes depending on the patient's condition. Patients can expect an increased need to urinate so they're encouraged to drink plenty of water following a session to replace fluids mobilized by the treatment.

In all cases it is a very specialized type of massage that should only be given by a trained therapist. For practitioners see http://www.lymphnet.org/resourceGuide/manualDrainage.htm

However once you've been properly taught the techniques you can perform a simplified version of MLD on yourself called **Simple Lymphatic Drainage** (SLD).

A more recent style of treatment was developed by French physician Dr. Bruno Chikly as a direct result of his award-winning research on the lymphatic system. **Lymph Drainage Therapy** (LDT) adds a new level of precision to traditional techniques. Therapists use all of their fingers with a flat hand to simulate gentle, wave-like motions with specific movements. Therapists are able to activate lymph and interstitial fluid circulation with these techniques and stimulate the immune and parasympathetic nervous systems.

As a type of massage therapy all practitioners must be licensed massage therapists. The US National Lymphedema Network cautions anyone taking anticoagulants, congestive heart patients and anyone else who may be sensitive to lymph movement. If you have any questions or concerns please check with your personal physician before beginning this type of therapy.

USER COMMENTS: *"Who knew that a lymph node could be so painful? These are things you didn't even know you had until somebody shows you how important they are to your health. Even an experienced massage therapist with a very light touch can get your attention when they first touch a node or collection/transmission spot and it's full or blocked. Ouch! What's really strange is that your whole body can be fine and just one spot can have a problem ... but it's a problem. The good news is that a good massage therapist can get things flowing again quickly and easily. Afterwards you feel lighter, more relaxed and just right again. It's funny how you may not notice that you're not feeling 100% until after you've had a massage with lymph drainage and then you feel 110%".*

"An experienced therapist can feel the fluids flow underneath their fingers so they can gently unblock the system and getting it moving again. Sometimes there may be little discomfort because the system is working well and the MLD is just sort of a flush. Other times part of is really needs the help. In any case it's a very beneficial process that helps the body maintain good health."

MASSAGE

www.amtamassage.org, www.abmp.com

A **Massage** is the process of applying pressure, tension, motion, or vibration to the soft tissues of the body. Working on the muscles, tendons, ligaments, joints, connective tissue or lymph system for a positive response can be done manually or with the aid of a device. In addition to just feeling wonderful it can be a form of therapy for parts of the body, or to the entire body, to help injuries heal, relieve stress, improve circulation or to help control pain. It is one of the oldest forms of therapy because it's been used by a variety of cultures for thousands of years.

According to the 2002 survey by the federal government 9.3% of those surveyed reported they'd had a massage at some time and 5.0% said they'd had a massage in the previous 12 months.

There are many different types of massage to choose from but there are several basic principles. First, good communication is essential to a beneficial massage. Client and massage therapist need to talk about what's expected before beginning the session. What areas need work or need to be avoided? How much pressure is comfortable? In addition the client's medical history and current physical condition need to be reviewed.

Depending on the type of massage it can involve the client lying on a massage table, sitting in a massage chair, or lying on a pad on the floor. In the U.S. clients are usually unclothed but draped with towels or sheet for warmth and privacy. The massage may be done beginning with the client facing up or down and then reversing for the second half of the session.

Below is a partial list of the different types of massage. Please note that the American Massage Therapy Association began the National Certification Exam in 1992. This exam is often used by states to regulate massage practitioners. Please check with your state's certification agency regarding local laws and regulations for massage therapists. Always remember to ask about your massage therapist's training and experience before beginning a massage.

USER COMMENTS: *"The massage experience totally depends on the therapist and what kind of massage you are getting at the moment. From my experience as a practitioner, every massage is a different experience, but always a totally relaxing moment. A massage can take you to Nirvana—to a place of ecstasy—that can totally relax the tension in the muscles. It is very important to drink water after a massage to help get rid of the toxins that the therapist has released. Some people get very relaxed after a massage but others get energized."*

Barefoot Deep Tissue

This technique is a combination of the barefoot styles of the Far East with Western bodywork. Clients normally lie on a floor mat, possibly with pillows or bolsters, and remain clothed. Sessions may last only a few minutes or more than an hour depending on the client's needs and condition. No oil is used because only a small area is worked on at one time. As a result of the therapist being able to apply a wide range of pressure very easily they're able to concentrate more closely on sensing the condition of the tissue being massaged for a more effective treatment. John Harris developed this modality as a deep tissue massage and for working on trigger points regardless of the size of the client.

Chair Massage or Corporate Massage

Perhaps one of the most convenient forms of massage, this technique is done with the client sitting in a special massage chair fully clothed but with restrictions like ties loosened for comfort. This technique focuses on the back, shoulders, neck and arms. Designed to relieve stress and promote circulation it normally lasts less than 25 minutes.

USER COMMENTS: *"This is one of the most wonderful innovations for trade shows and conventions! After standing or walking around all day on the* *concrete floors of a convention hall, this quick massage can save your back, your legs and your whole body. No wonder there are usually long lines waiting for a chair massage!"*

"My office has been using chair massage services for over a year and a half now and all we can say is we are ALWAYS looking forward to it! I personally would go crazy if we didn't have her here in our office at least once a month. My wish would be to have her here daily...but that's for the company to decide."

Deep Tissue Massage

This type of massage is often used to focus on a specific problem area. The massage therapist begins with a light, easy pressure and then works slowly into the depth of the muscle or soft tissues with gradually increasing pressure. Muscles may tighten if pressure is applied too deeply or quickly, possibly even causing damage, so it's important for the process to be slow and gradual with the comfort of the client in mind. Very little lubricant is used with this technique since it is focused in one small area at a time.

Erotic Massage or Tantra Massage

A very personal type of massage focusing on the genitals to stimulate blood flow and arousal, normally practiced by the sexual partner using self-help training materials.

Foot Massage

This localized form of massage uses several different types of motions. Stroking stimulates the blood vessels in the feet and promotes gentle warmth. A slow, easy rotation of the ankle is done to release stress and tension. Pivoting is done by the practitioner using their thumb to rub the toe joint on the bottom of the foot which can wiggle the toe. Toe Pulls are simply a gentle pulling motion applied to each toe which can pop the joint. Kneading the bottom of the foot is often done with the practitioner's fist. A technique called Finger Walking is simply rubbing one spot, usually with the thumb, and then moving a little horizontally to the next spot, and the next, etc.

Indian Head Massage

Indian men and women have practiced a type of massage based on the Ayurvedic healing system for thousands of years to stimulate circulation and relieve tension. It's believed that when the scalp is loose blood flows more freely to feed the hair root in order to prevent hair loss. There are many different techniques but Narenda Mehta developed the **Champissage** style in the 1970s while in London studying to become a physiotherapist. His massage technique involves the head but also the neck, shoulders and back for a more thorough procedure.
http://www.indianchampissage.com/

Lomilomi Massage

Lomilomi is an ancient form of healing art from Hawaii. Legends say that students were said to study for more than 20 years and received their final instructions from their master on his death bed. There are many different styles of Lomilomi, usually based on where it was developed.

Muscle Energy Technique (MET)

Dr. Fred Mitchell, Sr. developed this process in the early 1960s as a comprehensive manual therapy system but today it is almost an umbrella term for a wide range of muscle relaxation or stretching techniques. Two fundamentals of this process are reciprocal inhibition (RI) and post-isometric relaxation (PIR). RI is the response when the therapist uses a client's muscle to stretch the opposing muscle. PIR is the relaxation response that follows when an isometric contraction is released. This form of massage can be used as a sports massage. See www.muscleenergytechnique.com MET

Myofascial Release (also see Myofascial Release listing)

Myofascial Release refers to the manual soft tissue manipulation techniques for stretching the fascia and releasing bonds between fascia and integument, muscles, and bones, with the goal of eliminating pain, increasing range of motion and balancing the body. Injuries, stress, trauma, overuse and poor posture can cause restriction to fascia. Myofascial release frees fascial restrictions, and allows the muscles to move efficiently. This is usually done by applying shear, compression or tension in various directions, or by skin rolling. There are two main schools of myofascial release: direct and indirect methods.

Petrissage Massage

Petrissage is one of the five basic strokes of a Swedish massage. It's a kneading movement performed with the whole palm or finger tips by wringing, skin rolling, compression and lifting vertically on the muscle tissue. Often useful for warming of tissue for deeper work it increases circulation, softens superficial fascia and decreases muscle tension.

Shantala Massage

This type of ancient Indian technique is used to massage babies and children. It was introduced to the West by French obstetrician Dr. Frederique Leboyer and is described as a very simple technique. Its rhythmic movements help a child to relax, enhances their sense of security, sleep patterns and immune system. See www.ShantalaMassage.org

Shiatsu

From the Japanese words meaning "finger" and "pressure" the fundamental concept of Shiatsu is diagnosis and therapy combined to correct imbalances in the body. The technique uses mainly the thumbs but also finger pressure or pressure from the palm of the hand to work all along the meridians of the body. The focus is on treating the entire meridian but effective points may also be used. Normally the client is fully clothed on a floor mat for this work. Tokujiro Namiloshi founded the Japan Shiatsu College in 1940 to standardize Shiatsu Therapy. It is used around the world for promoting health and aiding in the healing of illness. (see Asian Bodywork listing.)

There are different types of Shiatsu such as the *Five Element Shiatsu* method which uses four examinations to determine the best massage pattern to harmonize the body. It uses the paradigm of the five elements to modify or control patterns of disharmony.

Interactive Eclectic Shiatsu combines traditional Japanese Shiatsu techniques with Traditional Chinese Medicine and Western-style soft tissue manipulation methods. It also uses dietary and herbal features for a comprehensive treatment style.

Myofascial Trigger Point Therapy or Trigger Point Therapy

MTPT is a massage style to relieve pain and restricted motion. Trigger points are painful points in muscles which cause the surrounding fascia to shorten and become tight. Direct or indirect pressure on trigger points causes them to unwind. This technique is used by a wide range of therapists ranging from doctors to chiropractors to massage therapists. See also *Myofacial Release* and www.MyofascialTherapy.org

Neuromuscular Massage

Therapy usually used to treat muscle spasm. Using the fingers, knuckles or elbow alternating levels of pressure are used but remaining constant for ten to thirty seconds at each pressure level.

Russian Clinical Massage

Russian Clinical Massage (RCM), also known as Russian Curative Massage is a cross-fiber technique with three distinct sections and 40+ movements. The first phase is slow for relaxation followed by the second fast and deep phase for therapeutic effect and then the slow third stage for relaxation and completion. The first massage school in Russia opened in the 17th century but the latest developments are claimed to reverse atrophy in muscles. The wide variety of techniques creates specific responses in the nervous system to speed up elimination of waste in the tissues, increase cell metabolism and recovery.

Sports Massage

The purpose of Sports Massage is to prepare an athlete for peak performance, and afterwards to relieve fatigue, swelling and muscle tension to prevent injuries and promote flexibility. Complete workouts today include caring for the wear-and-tear that comes with exercise. Since each sport uses different muscles in different ways the massage therapist must customize the Sports Massage to each athlete. Normally this will involve a combination of massage techniques including Swedish and Shiatsu along with deep tissue, trigger point work and acupressure.

Stone Massage

This method uses hot or cold stones, usually of basalt or marble, to massage the body. Stone sizes may vary from pebble to palm-sized and they may be placed directly on the skin or on a towel. They are usually placed on key energy points like energy meridians or chakras to improve energy flow. Depending on the technique the arrangement of stones may be in a straight line, dual lines similar to a cupping pattern in Traditional Chinese Medicine or other design. Using hot stones to give a deep massage creates a sensation of warmth while the heat relaxes the muscles and calms the nervous system. Hot stones also expand the blood vessels which help to push blood and waste through the body. It also allows for greater intensity than a regular massage.

When the client is suffering from any type of inflammation frozen or cooling stones are used to massage the body. In some cases both types of stones are used to stimulate the enlarging and then constricting of blood vessels for cleansing and healing.

Swedish Massage

The standard form of massage in the U.S. is the Swedish Massage which uses long, flowing strokes, often in the direction of the heart, to increase circulation and blood flow. There are six basic strokes which are applied with oil, cream or lotion to minimize the friction caused by a wider area of treatment. The types of strokes are effleurage, petrisage, friction, tapotement, compression and vibration. The approach was standardized by Dutch practitioner Johan Georg Mezger in the late 1800s.

USER COMMENTS: *"After doing four sessions last week, I felt better than I've felt in my adult life; more energized, joyous, and whole! It's hard to explain as I don't ever remember feeling this way, better circulation and so alive."*

Thai massage

This style is based on the Ayurveda system which originated in India. Clients lie on a floor mat in loose, comfortable clothing while the practitioner puts the body into many yoga positions. The practitioner leans on the client using hands and forearms to apply firm, rhythmic pressure to the body. The two-hour process usually follows energy meridians called Sen Lines which are similar to TCM meridians.

Tui na

In Chinese the words mean "push-grasp" which describes this acupressure treatment used to bring the client's body back into balance. The massage therapist may brush, knead, press or rub the areas between each of the joints called the eight gates to get the chi energy moving again in the meridians and muscles. The therapist will use range of motion technique along with traction, massage and the stimulation of acupressure points based on the Eight Principles. It is a form of Chinese manipulative therapy and part of Traditional Chinese Medicine so it may be used with other elements of TCM.

MYOFASCIAL RELEASE

www.myofascialrelease.com

Myofascial Release is a technique of sustained pressure for eliminating pain and increasing the body's range of motion. Dr. Janet Travell began using the term "Myofascial Trigger Point" in 1976 and the technique is also known as **Myofascial Trigger Point Therapy**

The fascia system is a single network of coverings on muscles, bones and organs that runs from head to foot connecting every part of the body. Its normal healthy condition is relaxed with the ability to stretch and move. When muscles are injured, stressed or inflamed their fibers and the surrounding fascia become short and tight, a condition which can spread to other locations in the body restricting motion and causing discomfort.

Practitioners using the direct method or deep tissue work use their knuckles, elbows or tools with sufficient pressure to slowly sink into the constricted fascia to stretch the fibers, allowing the tissue to reorganize into a more flexible manner.

A more gentle approach using lighter pressure is called the indirect method. This employs a stretching motion to allow the fascia to release or unwind itself. This technique uses the body's natural ability for self correction which often produces increased blood flow to the area and warmth.

The John F. Barnes' Myofascial Release Approach seminars are one source for this type of specialized training. There are also seminars are also available to learn how to use this technique to treat yourself.

USER COMMENTS: *"My injury was three years old and I had spent over $30,000 when I arrived at the John F. Barnes Myofascial Release Treatment Center. It was my last resort. The program that I went through changed my life. After only seven days at the John F. Barnes Myofascial Release Treatment Center, I was able to turn my neck around in circles."*

"Even though I was receiving good, traditional therapy, I continued to lose strength and functional mobility in my arms and shoulders. I was desperately discouraged and always in significant pain. Once I started receiving comprehensive therapy through the John F. Barnes Myofascial Release Treatment Center, I made more progress in two weeks than I had in the previous year. The therapists also helped me set up a home exercise program so I could continue to improve and have a more functional, pain free life."

NAMBUDRIPDAD ALLERGY ELIMINATION TECHNIQUE (NAET)
www.naet.com/

The **Nambudripad Allergy Elimination Technique** (NAET) was developed by Dr. Devi S. Nambudripad, M.D., D.C., Lac, PhD. (Acu.) in 1983. As a California acupuncturist, chiropractor and kinesiologist she created the natural, drugless, non-invasive process to deal with allergies and their health consequences.

NAET eliminates allergies using a combination of muscle testing, selective energy balancing using acupuncture or acupressure, nutrition, chiropractic techniques and traditional medicine. Neuromuscular Sensitivity Testing (NST) uses straight arm kinesiology techniques to evaluate the relative strength and weakness of the body's reaction to different substances. Following diagnosis one allergen is treated at a time in a specific sequence. In many cases a single treatment may successfully treat an allergen. An average person may have 15-20 food and environmental allergens which would require 15-20 office visits.

Training and certification in the technique is done by Dr. Nambudripad in basic and advanced seminars. Many NAET practitioners are chiropractors or acupuncturists.

USER COMMENTS: *"I almost lost my life. I was suffering from Crohn's disease. In and out of the hospital—and as every Crohn's patient discovers—treatment (other than surgical interventions), becomes large doses of prednisone (steroids) or other immuno-suppressant drugs. NAET saved my life, treatments addressed the CAUSE of Crohn's disease. My ongoing struggle to lower the dosage of prednisone was frustrated at 35 mg. Then, after just a few treatments of NAET, to handle the vicious food allergies, I was able to drop the dose from 35 mg to 10 mg WITH NO ADVERSE AFFECTS. There were no excessive symptoms of bleeding or starvation or relapse of the disease."*

"Ten months ago, I injured my shoulder when I was lifting with my trainer. Over the course of the following nine months, I tried a multitude of things to heal my shoulder. Not only did the above endeavors fail, my shoulder continued to have less and less mobility. After going through the first five NAET treatments, you tested me for acrylic nails. WOW! I tested a definite yes for the nails causing my shoulder impingement! Little did I expect such amazing results so quickly after my acrylic treatment. Within two weeks I had fifty percent mobility in my shoulder. Within four weeks I am at ninety-five percent improved. I am sure that last five percent will soon improve with a few laser treatments you have planned. My trainer was in amazement at the fast improvement. Obviously, NAET works!"

"From my experience, doctors are rushed and unable to explain things properly. They tend to offer medication rather than finding out the real source of 'why' you are in the state that you are in. There are a lot of answers out there, but that it's always going to be up to us to sift through it all and find what

works best. In my search of alternative therapies and treatments, I discovered a NAET practitioner. She has been a huge help and inspiration to me along the way and has already cleared me of a few of the many allergies that I have.

One of my most stubborn allergies to date has been an allergy to cats. Normally I couldn't spend more than 5 minutes near a cat before starting to experience wheezing, shortness of breath, and just basically felt miserable. The symptoms lasted far after leaving where the cats were and honestly it was a huge inconvenience in my life. After two treatments I can proudly state that I'm officially cleared of the cat allergy. Wow... what a blessing this has been!"

NETWORK SPINAL ANALYSIS™ CARE (NSA)

www.associationfornetworkcare.com

Network Spinal Analysis™ Care is a networking of different chiropractic techniques using gentle, specific touches in a consistent sequence to produce healing waves of relaxation. Developed in 1982 by New York chiropractor Dr. Donald Epstein the process enables chiropractors to release large amounts of spinal tension from patients.

By using light touch to the spine the patient's body learns to release patterns of tension, resulting in even deeper tensions being released. The finger or light hand contact is applied to specific access points along the neck and lower spine called spinal gateways which produces two waves of healing. The first is a breathing wave which releases immediate tension throughout the body to relax the patient. The second wave is a body-mind wave (or somatopsychic) which corresponds to the relaxing motion of the spine.

As you probably already know the spine is a string of bones sitting one on top of the other with pads called discs in between each one. Each vertebra has a hole, the spinal canal, where the spinal cord runs from the base of your brain to your tail bone. The connective tissues which attach this whole system to the body respond to all of the stresses and tensions of your life which impacts the functioning of your body. Using NSA to release tension and retrain the body how to release tension, patients become more peaceful and at ease with their life. This enhancement improves healing capacity and wellness.

USER COMMENTS: *"As a complete non-believer who'd never even gone to a chiropractor you can imagine how bad the pain in my neck was to get me to try NSA, but a good friend said it was very effective even if it was a little strange. She said it was more like touching than a regular chiropractic adjustment. He talked with me before the first session to get my medical history and then had me lay down on the massage table. He did some gentle touch around my back and then did this motion with his thumb at the bottom of my spine. Afterwards he stepped away for a few minutes so he could watch my breathing to see the blockages and then he worked on the other side of my back. He warned me that I might feel a little light headed and to get up slowly, and he was right.*

"My co-workers noticed a major change in my attitude after just the first session although it took several more visits to really deal with the stress. Things just didn't bother me the same way and I deal with problems more effectively.

"Some sessions I'd cry and other sessions I'd laugh but the therapist said it was all very normal and natural, I was simply releasing a lot of locked up emotions which were causing me stress. Best of all the neck pain completely disappeared and I've found a greater sense of calm and peace."

NEUROMODULATION TECHNIQUE (NMT)

www.NeuroModulationTechnique.com

The **NeuroModulation Technique**, or NMT, or the **Feinberg Technique** is based on muscle testing to access the body's control mechanisms to restore its ability to heal. It was developed in 2002 by Dr. Leslie S. Feinberg as the result of 20 years of energetic therapy research and his chiropractic experience, combining Western science with energy medicine.

The process uses muscle testing to communicate with the body's healing system. It uses active muscle testing (*see Applied Kinesiology listing*) along with passive muscle testing which is observing the response by the shortening or lengthening of a leg or arm. The process sequence first accesses the body's system to measure the errors causing the problem and finally to correct the situation by restoring the control system to normal operation.

Normally the patient is seated on a backless swivel chair so the practitioner can muscle test and treat easily. After each step the patient uses patterned breathing while the practitioner uses a special FDA approved device to stimulate vertebra with gentle taps. There may be variations of technique by practitioners depending on the situation.

Following an initial examination a practitioner will report the findings and discuss a reasonable schedule for improvement. Frequently it will take six to twelve sessions to reach the desired treatment milestones but since every individual and condition are unique, the results can vary.

Dr. Feinberg trains every NMT practitioner in his technique.

NUTRITION

www.nutrition.govn or www.nutrition.org, or,

http://www.eatright.org/cps/rde/xchg/ada/hs.xsl/index.html

There are literally hundreds of books available about diets and supplements so I've chosen to skip this topic. The main reason is that I'm just as confused as everyone else. There are diets from Atkins to Zone and everything in between, each with its own philosophy and supporting research. While I heartily agree that proper nutrition is a vital part of every health program I'm leaving this research to you.

The field of supplements is even more confusing. There are books devoted strictly to supplements that are several inches thick. Again, you'll have to figure this one out on your own but I'll at least give you a place to start:
      http://dietary-supplements.info.nih.gov/ or
http://www.cfsan.fda.gov/~dms/supplmnt.html

ORNISH PROGRAM

www.ornish.com

The **Ornish Program** can stop and even reverse heart disease without drugs or surgery. His best selling book "Dr. Dean Ornish's Program For Reversing Heart Disease" was first published in 1990 presenting scientific evidence on the success of his 4-step program. In it Dr. Eugene Braunwald, the chief of medicine at Harvard Medical School, was quoted on his reaction after he watched the PBS special on The Ornish Program. Dr. Braunwald said "Dr. Ornish's study is scientifically valid but it'll never play in Peoria." This statement reflects the attitude of many in the mainstream medical community which is why this program is included as a complimentary or alternative therapy.

Dr. Ornish began to question the fundamental premise of heart therapy at the very beginning of his medical career. He asked what would be the difference if patients changed the underlying cause of their heart problems instead of merely treating the symptoms with drugs and surgery. While insurance companies would gladly pay $50,000 for a heart by-pass operation or $5,000 to implant a stent to open an artery they couldn't see the benefit in spending a dime on prevention. This short-sighted approach has improved slightly but the insurance industry still has not sufficiently embraced the concepts of prevention.

The first step Dr. Ornish recommends is to quit smoking. For anyone with heart problems this step is abundantly clear in this day and age and does not require further explanation.

The special diet he recommends is very restrictive because that is what it takes to reverse heart disease. Losing weight can be done simply by eating less fat and fewer simple carbohydrates but reversing heart disease requires a radical change in diet to a vegetarian program balanced for proper nutrition.

Emotional stress is a key factor in this program because stress makes arteries constrict and blood clot faster which can lead to a heart attack. Stress management in the program involves yoga stretching, relaxation breathing techniques, meditation and guided imagery along with support groups. Sharing and connecting with other people can have a profoundly beneficial effect on stress.

The last part of the program is an extension of the emotional factor, it involves love and intimacy. Studies have shown that who are lonely and depressed are more likely to get sick than those who have a strong family connections, deep personal relationships and active participation in their community.

Dr. Ornish asks heart patients a simple question: How much do you want to live? If they are willing to make all of the necessary changes to their lives then their heart disease can be reversed.

USER COMMENTS: *"I was scared. Lying in bed in the still of the night my heart didn't sound like it had for the previous 55 years of my life. The beat was irregular, it not only sounded funny, it also felt strange. Weeks of tests labeled the condition an electrical problem, not a blockage but I wasn't going to take any chances with my life. Diet, exercise and any other changes that I had to make got made … quickly. Fear is a powerful motivator for change!*

The Ornish diet program is a tough change for a meat-and-potatoes guy. I probably had more vegetables in the first month on the program than I've had in the last year (or more)! Some of the recipes weren't too bad, they were modifications of foods I was already used to, but some were pretty strange.

Most of us never find the time to exercise but when your life depends on it, it's amazing how fast it becomes the #1 priority! Have to admit I was in pretty sad shape when I started but months into the program the results are starting to show. Meditation took some real dedication in the beginning but you can get used to it pretty quickly.

All in all, it's clear the program really does work. In the first month my triglycerides dropped by 1/3 and my total cholesterol level dropped into the normal range for the first time in my life. I'm happier, healthier and have more joy in my life than ever before so now I'm a walking testimonial for The Ornish Program."

OZONE THERAPY

www.ozoneuniversity.com

Ozone Therapy is a healing treatment that introduces ozone into the body. All 30 or so **oxygen therapies**, including ozone therapy, flood the body with single atoms (oxygen is O^2 and ozone is O^3). By putting large quantities of ozone into the body the single oxygen molecule that is unattached circulates freely to attack a wide range of illness and disease. It is considered to be anti-viral, anti-bacterial, anti-fungal because these organisms cannot live in an oxygen-rich environment. It is also said to have antioxidant stimulating capabilities.

This process normally uses an oxygen generator connected with an ozone generator to produce precisely controlled amounts of ozone. It may be introduced into the body in a variety of ways including:

1) Ingestion: drinking water or consuming olive oil that has been infused with ozone.
2) Rectal Insufflation: introducing ozone through the colon.
3) Vaginal Insufflation: introducing ozone into the female body.

4) Insertion in the Ear: placing the tube directly into the ear.
5) Transdermal (or through the skin): using a variety of methods including a baths, body suit, wraps or bagging, and other techniques.
6) Injection: placing ozone directly into the body in specially-prepared fluids, sometimes directly into a tumor site.
7) Inhalation: breathing in ozone directly, often using a sauna.

As an example, rectal insufflation is done by inserting the delivery tube directly into the colon so that humidified ozone can be absorbed directly into the bloodstream. If the large intestine is lined with debris the absorption rate is decreased. Treatments vary but often the first week normally uses a 30-second session for one to three days.

In America the first use of ozone therapy was by Dr. John H. Kellogg at his Battle Creek, Michigan sanitarium using ozone steam saunas in 1880. Since that time ozone therapy has been recognized in several countries around the world as an effective healing therapy.

Two of the most popular books are *Oxygen Therapies: A New Way of Approaching Disease* by Ed McCabe (1988) and his latest work *Flood Your Body With Oxygen* (2002).

The International Association for Oxygen Therapy was founded in 1972 to promote the use of ozone and other oxygen therapies. In the U.S. ozone therapy is usually taught privately or in naturopathic schools so it is wise to check the training and qualifications along with state regulations before beginning this type of therapy.

USER COMMENTS: *"I cured my asthma with the attachment where you breathe the ozone through olive oil. My asthma had been so bad that I couldn't even lie down when I slept and my MD had me on massive doses of steroids (which I stopped to do this therapy). It took five months, but I have remained asthma free with only occasional maintenance touch ups. An unexpected benefit to the treatment was that my eyesight improved."*

PLACEBO EFFECT

http://www.pbs.org/wgbh/pages/frontline/shows/altmed/snake/placebo.html

The **Placebo Effect** comes from the Latin phrase "I shall please" and it is used to describe the body's ability to heal itself. This completely natural type of healing should be the goal of every person since this type of healing has no side effects and no toxic chemicals. One of the first research reports on the process *The Powerful Placebo* (1955) and it concluded that an average of 32% of patients responded to the placebo.

Research today with the newest technology is unlocking many of the secrets of the placebo effect but it's also creating even more questions about this powerful human ability. Researchers in Italy have discovered that there isn't one placebo effect but many different types. Researchers in the U.S. have found that the process isn't simply a psychological phenomenon as originally thought but is a real, physical response to belief and expectation. Neuroscientist Helen Mayberg discovered in 2002 that inert pills (placebos) work the same way on brains of depressed people as antidepressants. Activity in the seat of higher thought, the frontal cortex, increased while activity in the area for emotions, the limbic regions, decreased.

Anatomy of Hope (2003) by Harvard Medical School physician Jerome Groopman, M.D. says that "A change of mind-set can alter neurochemistry both in a laboratory setting and in the clinic." Dr. Groopman experienced the power of the placebo effect releasing the brain's endorphins and enkephlins to relieve his own back pain.

The Allen Brain Atlas was completed in 2006. Founded by Microsoft co-founder Paul Allen, the project researched where each gene was activated in a mouse's brain because of its many similarities to human brains. They discovered that 80% of the 21,000 genes in a mouse body were activated in the brain, more than anyone expected. This is a possible indication of the mind-body connection and the placebo effect.

Medically inactive pills, often called sugar pills, are used to simulate real medications during testing of new medications to determine if they're more effective than the placebo effect. If the new product can't produce positive results higher than the placebo then it will not be approved by the Food and Drug Administration (FDA). The pharmaceutical industry has successfully tainted the term "placebo effect" with a very negative connotation because to them it is a real problem. However it should be remember that the placebo effect is a powerful healing process. Because it can't be patented and sold for a profit this all-natural healing capacity has a negative effect on the modern drug industry but a very positive effect on everyone else.

Unfortunately for the drug industry the rate of positive responses to placebos have improved over the years as a result of better test design and the use of so-called active placebos which provide a detectable response unrelated to the problem. The better the placebo response the more difficult it is for new drugs to demonstrate effectiveness.

In June 2004, the FDA began changing from a single molecule (rifle shot) mentality to accepting the more holistic perspective of using whole compounds (shotgun approach). New guidelines were issued making it easier for companies to turn herbal remedies into Western medicines. The FDA even created a new botanical review team led by Jinhui Dou who was born in China and has a degree from the Beijing University of Chinese Medicine.

RAINDROP TECHNIQUE
www.younglivingworld.com/resources/raindrop_main.asp

The **Raindrop Technique** is a combination of aromatherapy, massage and reflexology designed to bring the body into structural and electrical alignment.

The 8-step process developed by Don Gary Young, N.D. and introduced in his book *Raindrop Technique* (2003).

The process was inspired by the healing practices of the Lakota Indians. It uses aromatic essential oils dropped like rain from a height of about six inches above the back and massaged into the back muscles along the vertebrae. Oils are also used to treat special locations on the feet in a modified form of reflexology. The process is reported to be particularly effective for abnormalities in the spine.

D. Gary Young is also the founder of the Young Living Essential Oils company.

USER COMMENTS: *"I have a daughter who struggled with a lot of achiness due to undiagnosed Lyme Disease for three years. Her main struggles were muscle aches and overall fatigue. I started using the Raindrop Technique® as described in the Essential Oils Desk Reference. Within ten minutes of using it, I have a symptom-free, energetic ten-year-old again"*

"I hurt my back in November 2004. I was in severe pain all day every day for months; sometimes it was excruciating. In June 2005, I started doing yoga, which helped, but I still felt bad pain. Then in August, I began having Raindrop Technique® done on me. Each time I have a treatment with the oils, I make a major leap forward—less pain and more mobility. By October I had a pain-free week. It is a real boon to be getting my life back. I am on the mend and expect to be completely well soon."

RELOX™ PROCEDURE

www.drrind.com

The **Relox**™ procedure is designed to help stroke victims recover function. The process combines nutrition and oxygen for synergy of the components. Nutritional therapy involves taking vitamins and minerals both orally and intravenously. At the same time patients are receiving oxygen by standard face mask technique.

In many cases **Hyperbaric Oxygen Therapy** *(see listing)* is also used as part of the therapy to magnify the effectiveness of the Relox™ procedure. This is the application of pure oxygen at higher than normal pressures. HBOT chambers were originally designed to help deep sea divers recover from a condition known as "the bends" resulting from insufficient decompression. Today the technique is used for a variety of conditions involving circulation problems.

The process was developed by Bruce Rind, M.D., a board certified anesthesiologist with both traditional and alternative training working in the Washington, D.C. area.

USER COMMENTS: *"Seven years ago, I injured my ankle. The pain and swelling were constant. I could barely walk. My orthopedist recommended fusing the bones, which he said would cause me to lose all ankle/foot motion.*

There was no guarantee the pain or swelling would go away. I decided to find an alternative to that approach. Dr. Rind treated my ankle with prolotherapy. After five treatments, all the pain and swelling were gone. Since then, I hike several miles daily on my farm. The pain has not returned since."

"I was in a near fatal car accident in 1997. I was in a coma for one month. When I came out of it, I couldn't move, speak or remember anyone I knew from before. After a few months my memory started to return and I began a rehabilitation program for speech and walking. Rehab lasted nine months. My speech was slurred, walking was difficult and I could walk ten feet per minute.

I remained this way until Relox therapy. Within one hour of the first treatment, my speech, walking, balance and short term memory all had visibly and dramatically improved. At first I thought I was dreaming. By the next day I realized that my life had changed in a very positive way. I received one more treatment which included osteopathic adjustment. After that treatment my walking improved noticeably."

ROLFING®
www.rolf.org or www.rolfguild.org

Rolfing® Structural Integration was created in the 1950s by Dr. Ida Pauline Rolf as a holistic system of soft tissue manipulation and movement education. It's a unique blend of function and structure enabling the body to work in proper alignment with gravity.

In 1920 Ida Rolf received her Ph.D. in biochemistry. As a result of her own and other's health issues she researched the problems of bones, muscles and movement. One of her popular quotes is "Some individuals may perceive their losing fight with gravity as a sharp pain in their back, others as the unflattering contour of their body, others as constant fatigue...They are off balance. They are at war with gravity."

Her study of Hatha Yoga influenced the development of Rolfing. She recognized that bodies which are properly aligned and functioning with gravity have less stress and pain with more energy, improved posture and body awareness. The legs are aligned to the hips, shoulders and rib cage with the body positioned correctly over the feet so that all of the joints are integrated to each other.

Rolfing begins with the Ten Series, a sequence of ten one-hour sessions with the patient lying down on a massage table. At times the client will be asked to walk back and forth to evaluate progress. Each session has a specific goal in the sequence. While the client is guided through each movement the Rolfer manipulates the fascia to restore it to its original length applying slow-moving pressure with their knuckles, thumbs, fingers, elbows and even knees. Working with the deep myofascial structures to separate layers and align muscles the process acquired a reputation for being painful in the

1960s. Today most Rolfers work closely with clients for comfort and effectiveness.

Following a period of time after the initial sessions many clients choose a tune-up series. There is also an Advanced Series of five sessions available. Today, many Rolfers also offer movement training to compliment the structural integration.

In 1989, a group of dedicated followers started the Guild for Structural Integration to maintain Ida Rolf's traditional work and "the Recipe". This group of educators and practitioners has its own training programs and certification standards for GSI practitioners.

The Rolf Institute of Structural Integration (RISI) also trains and certifies Rolfers and Rolf Movement Practitioners around the world. Practitioners in the U.S. must be licensed as massage therapists, please check your state agencies for requirements.

USER COMMENTS: *"Rolfing is about the good hurt, but after being all bent over and out of place, anything seems like an improvement. Actually, it IS a big improvement. Working with a 'gentle Rolfer' it didn't seem like there was a lot of movement going on, but man did it feel like the next day. Walking back and forth over and over felt like different people were doing the walking. After all of the Ten Series sessions it's amazing how grounded you feel, also taller, stronger and more coordinated. There is just a grace and flow after everything has been put back together again. I will admit that additional 'tune-up' sessions were needed but after more than 50 years of gravity it wasn't a big surprise."*

"I am sold on Rolfing because I get to do all the sports I want to even though I don't have a perfect back. Rolfing does not correct the inherent changes in my back, but it allows me to continue to do rigorous activities and makes me more aware of my body and helps with the pain, discomfort and stiffness. Rolfing gives me pain relief and keeps me symmetric so I can count on my body more."

"Massage offers immediate relief, but it's not lasting. Muscles endure repetitive strain. A simple injury with a suitcase can develop into a shoulder cramp, the muscle shortens from strain. Rolfing returns you to your optimum and balances your body. Chiropractic is like massage, it offers temporary relief, but you have to keep going back, the underlying problem is still there. Rolfing straightens out the underlying problem. It helps me with downhill and cross-country skiing, and bicycling which require balance. Having the body in balance supports my athletic interests."

TAI CHI or Tai Chi Chuan or T'ai Chi Ch'üan or Taijiquan
Website: http://nccam.nih.gov/health/taichi/
http://www.wustyle.com/en/index.html

Tai Chi is a soft style, or relaxed form, of martial art. It is based on the Yin/Yang concept of meeting hard with soft, using leverage rather than muscle tension to neutralize attacks. The easily recognizable, slow, gentle, flowing movements of Tai Chi have been seen in large crowds across China and around the world. It is often seen as a kind of moving meditation. It follows many of the principles of Traditional Chinese Medicine and has many reported health benefits, especially for the elderly. Researchers have found the long-term Tai Chi practice has favorable effects in balance, flexibility, cardiovascular fitness with reports of reduced pain, stress and anxiety in healthy subjects. It has also been shown to decrease falls in the elderly.

There are many different styles today but they're based on the system originally taught by the Chen family to the Yang family beginning in 1820. Training involves learning the solo routines called "forms". There is also advanced training known as "pushing hands" for two people and also weapons training. There are several major styles of Tai Chi, each named after the Chinese family where it originated. These are: Chen Style, Yang Style, Wu Style, Hao Style, Sun Style and Zhaobao Style. In 1956 the Chinese Sports Committee shortened the Yang Family form to 24 postures, often called the Short Form of Tai Chi. The longer traditional solo forms can have 88 to 108 postures. In 1976 a combination form called the Combined 48 Forms was created. Today there are dozens of new styles and hybrids which have grown out of the main styles.

In 1970 Taoist Tai Chi was introduced to the West by Master Moy Lin-Shin. This form is different because it is designed to promote and restore health. The Taoist Style uses greater stretching and turning in all of the movements to increase the benefits of Tai Chi.

There is no universal certification process for Tai Chi so almost anyone can call themselves a teacher. As with all exercise programs it is wise to first check with your physician and also carefully research the training and experience of the Tai Chi instructor.

USER COMMENTS: *"The first thought I had was "How hard can it be to learn 24 moves?" As it turns out, it can take a lifetime. An impatient American can learn the fundamentals of the moves in a few weeks or months but the subtleties, the wonderful delicate touches, can take many years.*

"I signed up for the class because I loved the grace of the movements and needed some serious stress reduction in my life. This moving meditation as it's called seemed idea. It looks easy but the effects are amazing. There is a feeling of peace and freedom after doing Tai Chi that is difficult to explain. It looks easy but it can feel like a workout when you're done, but it also relaxes the body and the mind in a unique way.

"For those of us with limited muscle memory it means practicing regularly or it's like starting all over again!"

TRAGER® APPROACH

www.trager.com or www.trager-us.org

The **Trager® Approach** uses gentle, natural movements to produce deep relaxation and increased physical mobility. Underlying physical and mental patterns which may have developed from accidents, illness or other trauma are also released with this process. It uses movement education for mind-body integration to produce long-lasting effects. Some people use this technique for personal growth. The approach had also been known as Trager Work or Trager Psychophysical Integration.

Dr. Milton Trager discovered the principles of his technique as a teenaged boxer when he intuitively accessed a style of bodywork while giving a rubdown to his trainer. Surprised by the experience he applied it to his father and after just two sessions managed to clear up his father's chronic sciatica. Dr. Trager spent the next 50 years refining and expanding his discovery to learn more about the effects of these gentle movements on the nervous system and the unconscious mind.

There are two different aspects of The Trager® Approach which complement each other. The first is a passive technique called tablework where the client is lying on a comfortable table. Before each session the trained practitioner enters into a meditative state called "hook up" to better communicate with the client's body. Then the practitioner supports and moves the client in normal ways but with a touch that provides the sensation of effortless motion. Sessions normally last 60 to 90 minutes and the client is dressed comfortably but with a minimum of clothing.

Mentastics® is the active portion of The Trager Approach®, taught in both private and group sessions. The instructions for these simple movements teach clients how to take care of themselves and relieve stress on their own during daily activities. These self-induced movements reinforce the quality of effortless movement developed during tablework.

The *Trager* Institute in 1980 and today the United States Trager Association's certification program requires at least 409 hours of training normally taking at least six months to complete.

USER COMMENTS: *"Trager® has been the most memorable and life-altering experience I have had in healthcare. From the ages of 19 through 30, I was consistently in physical pain, unable to be helped by various forms of treatment including cortisone treatments, muscle relaxers, chiropractic, massage, meditation and hypnosis. I was finally diagnosed with muscular rheumatism, told I would have to learn to relax and accept a slower lifestyle. I remember as if it was today, my third Trager Session... I stood up off the table, free of pain, with a sense of a new body. Like all people, I do experience occasional pain, but for the last 25 years, and today at 55, I live a very active lifestyle without daily pain. Thanks to that Trager session and the Trager exercises, Mentastics®, I can bring back the feelings of freedom, relax and know I am not trapped by pain. It is that freedom that led me to become a Trager Practitioner, helping my clients... and delighted to hear them say 'Trager is amazing, I don't have that pain anymore.'"*

"My chronic shoulder pain was treated with cortisone injections and with many physical therapy visits, but Trager® eliminated the pain and gave me more range of motion."

"I don't know that I've ever felt as relaxed as I was on your table. My memory of it is certainly like floating on a cloud. The residual effects have left me calmer and clearer. I had been having trouble relaxing, especially when it was time to do so. Since my session with you, I'm able to recall the feelings and sink in, allowing myself to rest onto that cloud. The Mentastics®, too, continue to help me practice relaxing my muscles. I can certainly see how successive sessions would build and reinforce the sensory memory."

TTOUCH-FOR-YOU

tteam-ttouch.com

TTouch-For-You is the therapeutic adaptation of the **Tellington Touch** animal therapy developed by Linda Tellington-Jones in 1983. The therapy was developed after training with Dr. Moshe Feldenkrais (see **Feldenkrais® Method**). While owners were learning the therapy for their animals they'd experiment on each other and the benefits for people were quickly obvious.

This is a system of circular motions, lifts and slides that works to activate the body's potential at the cellular level. There are twenty different types of TTouches including Ear TTouches, Hair Slides, Heart Tug and Octopus, often using small circular motions. One example is The Hair Pulling Slide technique that applies gentle pressure, moving in the direction away from the scalp to the ends of small sections of hair, which creates pressure at and beneath the scalp which is quite pleasurable. This relaxation may lower your pulse rate and blood pressure, slow respiration and neutralize stress chemicals in the body associated with the "fight or flight" response.

Linda Tellington-Jones co-authored *Massage And Physical Therapy For The Athletic Horse* based on the teachings of her grandfather, William Caywood. Her latest book is *The Ultimate Horse Behavior and Training Book.*

USER COMMENTS: *"I recently flew to Indiana for a week to be with my parents. My father is 88 years old and has Alzheimer's. He was talking gibberish. Not one word was intelligible, just a string of syllables. I put both hands on his bald head and begin Lying Leopard TTouches, very slowly. He was suddenly silent. For about 2 or 3 minutes, I continued all over his head. Then I sat down. He began talking in well-articulated words and sentences! My mom was amazed!"*

"A client of mine has found a way to reduce the most wearing symptoms of his Multiple Sclerosis to a minimum with Tellington-TTouch For You®. It has improved his quality of life significantly. He is still incurably ill but his worst symptoms have decreased so much that he has found a new interest in everything. He is also cheerful again—according to his wife he is almost the same person he was before the disease spread in his body. He himself confirms 'Today I enjoy life again!'"

"I fell 9-½ feet off a stair landing and landed on a concrete sidewalk on my left hip. I endured months of pain, limited mobility, side effects of pain pills and

a generally deteriorating quality of life. I felt like a piece of beef with little con-nectedness to my doctors or the physical therapist. When I first experienced a session of Tellington TTouch I was pretty desperate, experiencing a significant amount chronic pain, and in an emotionally dark and hopeless place.

"My first session was quite an amazing experience. For the first time in a year I actually felt good. I'm not sure how she knew where all the terribly pain-ful spots in my body were but she seemed to find all of them. I laid on the couch on my right side and she worked on my entire left side. My shoulder, back, hip, thigh, knee, shin, ankle and foot received gentle attention. My breathing became deep and relaxed and with every exhale I experienced pain leaving my battered left side. The feeling was such an immense relief from the searing pain I'd been enduring for a year that I felt 'high'. Most prominent however, was a sense of well-being I had forgotten could exist in my world. For the first time since my injury, I felt that maybe there could be hope for the relief of pain I had endured. I am not attempting to indicate I've had a miraculous recovery with Tellington TTouch. I want to articulate the treatments have significant therapeutic efficacy and combined with medical interventions the sessions provided a degree of progress and hope of getting well I had not achieved in a year."

"Our TTouch session was not like any other type of body work I have re-ceived. I appreciated how much you checked in with how I felt as you worked with me. It helped me to understand that TTouch is really something you do WITH the person, not just TO them. While I felt relaxed after our session, I also felt energized and decided to go out for a walk. I was surprised that I felt good enough to climb up and down a very long flight of stairs at my local park and still my knee felt great. My knee hasn't felt that good since I injured it. Thank you for the time you spent with me. I'd like to schedule another session as much for the feeling of calm well being I had as for the benefit of my knee."

WATSU® or Water Shiatsu
www.waba.edu

Watsu® therapy is one of the early forms of aquatic bodywork. It combines elements of shiatsu, muscle stretching, massage and dance with graceful, fluid movements in a warm water environment. Working in water requires the client be supported at all times which creates a connection between therapist and client that is much deeper than work done on a table. The therapeutic benefits of warm water include greater freedom of movement and deep relaxa-tion.

The technique was developed in 1980 by Harold Dull, a Northern Califor-nia massage therapist. After returning from Japan he began floating his **Zen Shiatsu** students in the warm water of Harbin Hot Springs. The idea of stretching to open the flow of energy channels is even older than acupunc-ture. Stretching also strengthens muscles and increases flexibility. The support provided by working in warm water relieves compression in joints like vertebrae and decreases muscle tension allowing movement that is not possible out of the water.

In addition to traditional Watsu® there are three major styles: **Waterdance**; **Healing Dance** and the **Jahara Technique**. The Waterdance technique is done completely beneath the surface. The Healing Dance style is a mix between regular Watsu and water dance. The Jahara Technique is called the gentlest form because of its constant support and gentle bodywork. One of the common features are moments of stillness alternated with rhythmical, flowing movements, often using the Water Breath Dance which is the rising and falling back caused by each breath. Originally Watsu® involved a therapist supporting the client but with the use of floatation devices today there is a greater range of movement possible. Sessions are usually 50-60 minutes but can vary depending on your therapist and condition.

Watsu® is practiced in more than 40 countries and is accepted as a key methodology in rehabilitation by aquatic therapists. The Worldwide Aquatic Bodywork Association (WABA) supervises Watsu® standards along with maintaining a registry of authorized practitioners. Since this is considered a type of massage, please check with your state regarding regulations and certifications in your area.

USER COMMENTS: *"You've never really been relaxed until you've had a Watsu session! After trying massage and even Rolfing, Watsu was recommended to help me relax so the muscles could heal better. Floating in warm water (in my case it happened to be saltwater for added buoyancy) while wearing floatation devices on my legs, arms and around my waist and head was a totally weightless sensation. It took a few minutes for me to actually relax and not worry about drowning but the calming words of the therapist helped guide me through the process.*

"The movements are slow and gentle and sometimes you can barely tell you're moving at all. Stretches start small and grow as your muscles adapt. There are motions possible floating in water that just can't be done on a massage table, and they're wonderful.

"The slow breathing and constant support of the therapist brought back memories of being cradled in my mother's arms as a baby. The relaxation that you feel after a Watsu session is incredible, like a massage and hot tub rolled together."

"The mother of an 11-year-old boy with ankylosing spondylitis (arthritis of the spine) witnessed that peace (from Watsu) in her pain-ridden child. The disease, which causes severe pain in the joints, was prevalent in the boy's back and hips. He was also diagnosed with attention deficit hyperactivity disorder (ADHD). getting treatments three to four times a week with Watsu seemed to reduce his negative behaviors, especially through the eyes of his mother, the nurses and staff."

YOGA

www.yogajournal.com

In the U.S. **yoga** is considered mainly a form of exercise concentrating on postures (asanas) and breathing. The rest of the world recognizes yoga as a means for both physical health and spiritual mastery. Yoga connects the movement of the body with the rhythm of the breath and the mind. According to the 2002 survey of CAM practices by the federal government 7.5% of Americans have ever used yoga and 5.1% used it in the previous 12 months. Yoga Journal's 2005 survey estimates there are 16.5 million yoga practitioners in the U.S. today.

Yoga is a collection of ancient spiritual practices originating in India for integrating mind, body and spirit to achieve oneness with the universe. While it is one of the schools of Hindu philosophy it is a spiritual practice, not a religion, and it does not require any specific beliefs for participation. Yoga is also central to Buddhism, Tibetan Buddhism, Jainism and has influenced many other religions.

A male who practices yoga is a yogi, and a female practitioner is a yogini. While there is a lot of crossover between yoga schools and variations within each style there are many common features. Hatha yoga is the most popular style in the U.S. today. It was introduced in the 15th century as an outgrowth of an older style known as Raja yoga. It's used to prepare the body for higher meditation. Because it develops health and flexibility, students in the U.S. are usually not interested in the complete Hatha yoga process which deals with spiritual development.

Hatha represents opposing energies such as hot and cold, male and female, in a similar fashion to the Chinese concept of yin and yang. It works to balance the mind and body by physical exercises called asanas using controlled breathing, and the calming of the mind through relaxation and meditation. These postures develop balance, strength and reduce stress.

The traditional instructions for Hatha yoga include having a glass of fresh water before the session. The asanas should be done on an empty stomach to prevent discomfort, and are best done in the early morning. Asanas should not involve force or pressure and movements should be slow and gentle. Breathing should always be done through the nose and in a controlled manner. Yoga should be done in a peaceful, clean, well-lit room that is well ventilated.

The following is a partial list of yoga styles.

Ananda yoga is a way to release unwanted tensions and to grow spiritually. This system uses silent affirmations while holding a posture, a technique intended to deepen and enhance the subtle benefits of each asana. This is a technique for aligning the body, its energy, and the mind with a series of gentle postures created to move energy upward to the brain. See www.expandinglight.org

Anusara Yoga® is said to mean, "stepping into the current of divine will." This new system developed by John Friend blends the human spirit with the science of biomechanics. It is different from other yoga systems by three features: Attitude; Alignment and Action. See www.anusara.com

Ashtanga yoga is a system of six, fast-paced series of sequential postures of increasing difficulty which is why sweating comes easy. See www.yogaworkshop.com

Bikram yoga is also called hot yoga because room temperatures can be near 100° Fahrenheit. This environment helps move toxins out of the body by sweating. There is a series of 26 traditional Hatha postures directed at each body system. See www.bikramyoga.com/

Hatha yoga is often a blending of different styles of yoga under what has become almost a generic banner. This being the case, it's probably a good idea to check into the class to see if it's more in the meditative or active style before signing up. It might not hurt to check into the teacher's training and experience too. http://www.abhidhyan.org/Teachings/Hatha_Yoga.htm

Integral yoga is the form of yoga Sri Swami Satchidananda developed in 1966 to help people integrate the teachings of yoga into their everyday life. This is to promote greater peace and tolerance in the individual. http://www.iyiny.org/Integral_Yoga_Institute/integral_yoga_institute.html

Integrative Yoga Therapy was introduced in 1993 in San Francisco by Joseph Le Page, M.A. This is a yoga teacher-training program designed specifically for medical environments such as hospitals and rehabilitation centers. See www.iytyogatherapy.com

Iyengar yoga puts an intense focus on the subtleties of each position by requiring students to hold each position longer. Students can pay close attention to the precise muscular and skeletal alignment this system demands with this longer attention. The system also uses props such as belts and chairs to deal with special needs such as injuries. See www.iyisf.org

Jivamukti yoga is a highly meditative form of yoga that is also physically challenging. Sessions may include chanting, meditation, readings, music, and affirmations along with the postures. See www.jivamuktiyoga.com

Kali Ray Tri Yoga® was created in 1980 as a new flowing method of yoga. Tri Yoga fundamentals include relaxation-in-action, wave-like spinal movements and economy of motion. With the systematic approach students can remain with Basics or progress to subsequent levels. Music accompanies the classes ending with meditation. See www.triyoga.com

Kundalini yoga was a secret process that came from the Tantra yoga path until Yogi Brahan introduced it to the West in 1969. It is supposed to help seekers of enlightenment from all religious paths tap into their greater potential. This system uses postures and dynamic breathing techniques along with chanting and meditating on mantras. Students focus on awakening the energy at the base of the spine and drawing it upward through each of the traditional seven chakras. See www.3HO.org.

Phoenix Rising Yoga Therapy is a synthesis of traditional yoga and contemporary body-mind psychology which can produce a release of physical tensions and emotional blocks. See www.pryt.com

Power yoga was a term Beryl Bender Birch created to describe Ashtanga yoga to Americans. It's a workout of a series of poses designed not to create heat and energy flow but to serve as a traditional methodology for spiritual transformation. Because of the athletic and powerful nature of the physical portion of the system it's popular in health clubs and gyms. See www.power-yoga.com

Sahara yoga is a method of meditation created in 1970 to bring a new level of awareness. The process is supposed to help you experience the power of the divine as your awareness expands. As a result students become more integrated and balanced, capable of effortless spiritual growth.

Sivananda Yoga is a path to learn about who you really are. It is supposed to help you appreciate each level of experience. www.sivananda.org

Svaroopa® yoga teaches different ways of doing familiar poses. It focuses on opening the spine by beginning at the tailbone and progressing through each area. This is a consciousness-oriented yoga that also promotes healing which many consider a very approachable style. See www.masteryoga.org

Tibetan Yoga is composed of five flowing movements. It is an active workout that features constant motion. Students may begin with 10 or 12 repetitions and work their way up to the 21 repetitions of the full routine. See www.nyingma.org

Viniyoga is a practice designed to work on all levels. The poses are synchronized with the breath. It is a process for developing a style to meet each person's needs as they grow. See www.viniyoga.com

White Lotus yoga is a flowing style that varies from gentle to vigorous depending on ability and comfort level. Classes involve alignment, breath, and the theories of yoga. See www.WhiteLotus.org

ZEN BODYTHERAPY® or Zentherapy®

www.zentherapy.org

Zentherapy® is the belief that life is the flow of energy called Ki or Chi. As we live and grow, this life-force energy shapes our emotions and bodies. Zentherapy® releases the changes caused by physical, psychological and spiritual traumas so the natural form of the body can return. By releasing the traumas held in the body, the mind and spirit also change.

William S. ("Dub") Leigh developed the process as a result of his studies with three masters. He learned about the structure of the body from Ida Rolf and about function from Moshe Feldenkrais. In Hawaii he trained under Zen Master and martial artist Tanouye Tenshin Rotaishi, a healer adept at the use of Ki. By combining the deep-tissue work of Rolfing®, the body re-education of the Feldenkrais Method® along with the energy training of Tanouye Rotaishi, he created a unique new process.

The International Zentherapy® Institute, Inc. is headquartered in Hawaii and is the only source for training and certification in this modality. As a form of bodywork, practitioners must have massage licensing in most states.

BODY DEVICES

COLD LASER THERAPY or Low Level Laser Therapy (LLLT) or Cold Laser Acupuncture

http://en.wikipedia.org/wiki/Laser_therapy

The use of light for healing goes back thousands of years but the process is growing in popularity with the latest technology. Light or photon energy with limited power, a few J/cm2 with laser power of 50 mW or less, penetrates up to two inches below the surface of the skin with no tissue damage. There is no heat or pain from this type of device and it is being used to treat a variety of health problems.

The FDA first approved the use of **cold laser therapy** to treat neck and shoulder pain, following with approval for carpal tunnel syndrome in 2002, however most insurance companies deny coverage considering the technology experimental. These devices are also being used to treat a variety of inflamed conditions of soft tissues and joints such as sports injuries, arthritis, back pain and other injuries to the musculoskeletal system. Cold lasers are even being used as "pointless" acupuncture, using light energy to stimulate the acupuncture points without pain and to stimulate lymph drainage. One of the most popular cold laser acupuncture treatments is to help stop smoking. Cold lasers are even being used to stimulate hair follicles to prevent hair loss and promote hair growth.

USER COMMENTS: *"This (cold laser) unit has been an invaluable tool in helping us treat our veteran patients who suffer from chronic pain and chronic non-healing ulcers. Before we had this unit, we were treating chronic pain patients with regular processes including moist heat, TENS and microcurrent. We have had moderate success in reducing patients' pain with these processes. With the unit we have had significant reduction in pain levels when treating our chronic pain patients. We have had some patients' pain levels decrease to almost zero (on a 10-point scale) after one or two treatments. This includes patients with such painful conditions as diabetic neuropathy and dry gangrene."*

"I have been in practice for over 35 years working in the field of head, neck and facial pain. There is no question in my mind that this laser is the one and only modality that a physical therapist needs in his tool box."

"Too often we think that what we can't see won't hurt us. Wrong! While going through physical therapy for a back injury, the therapist decided to use a cold laser treatment to promote healing. There was a chart on the wall of what points they're supposed to use, but apparently she had decided that since it was "painless" that it would be okay to just run it all up and down the back muscles to stimulate healing.

"It also stimulated every acupuncture point in my back! The result was that I didn't sleep for nearly two days because my system was pumped full of adrenaline and stimulated. At this point everyone really needs to learn about the specific machine being used, the training the operator has had, their results (and problems) and be very, very careful."

HYPERBARIC OXYGEN THERAPY (HBOT)

www.hyperbaricmedicalassociation.org or www.hbot.com

Hyperbaric Oxygen Therapy or HBOT refers to treating the body with 100% oxygen at higher than normal pressure. The term comes from "hyper" meaning increased and "baric" which relates to pressure. Normally we breathe 20% oxygen at one atmospheric absolute, which is abbreviated as ATA. With HBOT pure oxygen is given at up to two times normal pressure either in an individual or group chamber. This combination of increased oxygen and pressure results in pushing oxygen for healing into the blood, fluids and body tissues at up to twenty times normal levels.

Originally the technique was developed to help skin divers recover from surfacing too quickly, a condition known as "the bends", but the benefits of HBOT have been demonstrated on a wide variety of health problems. Pressurized oxygen has been especially beneficial for neurological problems such as cerebral palsy, brain injury, Multiple Sclerosis and stroke. HBOT has also been used successfully to treat peripheral vascular disease, burns, diabetic ulcers, carbon monoxide poisoning and macular degeneration. HBOT can help restore function and increase healing whenever blood flow and oxygen delivery has been compromised. Treatments usually last between an hour to an hour-and-a-half but 50 to 100 treatments may be required for full effect.

While accepted by many in the mainstream medical community the therapy is not widely used, possibly due lack of physician familiarity. It's estimated that less than 20% of the medical schools in the country have their own hyperbaric oxygen facility and perhaps only 15% or 20% more may have access to one. Simply put, if doctors aren't trained or don't know about a therapy then they're reluctant to prescribe it. This chicken-and-egg situation is a common problem with complimentary and alternative therapies.

The cost for a single HBOT treatment session may vary from $150 to nearly $1,000 per hour. Medicare did approve HBOT for the treatment of diabetic foot wounds in 2003 but most insurance companies deny coverage because the FDA has not issued a formal approval due to a lack of research. It costs millions of dollars to conduct the necessary research for FDA approval but since oxygen can't be patented the profit potential is limited. Without FDA approval and subsequent insurance reimbursement there is limited interest in developing new HBOT facilities. This is a common problem with CAM therapies.

LIGHT THERAPY or Phototherapy
www.mayoclinic.com/health/seasonal-affective-disorder/DS00195

Light Therapy or **phototherapy** is normally associated with treatment of a particular type of depression known as **seasonal affective disorder** or SAD, also called winter depression. Exposure to bright lights reduces the brain's production of melatonin which controls the body's internal clock, reducing the effects of SAD. Recommendations are for at least two hours of sunlight each day for good physical and emotional health.

Treatment is done with special fixtures which produce bright light, normally up to twenty times light levels in an office or home. Originally full-spectrum bulbs were used because they most closely resembled natural light but some research suggests that brightness is more important than color spectrum. Treatment products produce light ranging from 2,500 to 10,000 lux and exposure times will vary from up to two hours with lower power units to approximately 30 minutes with high-powered devices. Exposure is usually recommended first thing in the morning to help reset the body's clock to a spring day. While light therapy may be used in the evening for severe cases, it can also interfere with normal sleep patterns. Clocks which mimic normal sunrise, called Dawn Clocks, are also used to treat SAD.

Light Therapy is also used to treat jet lag since it can be useful in resetting the body's clock. Other types of light therapy are used to treat acne, psoriasis and eczema. Full-spectrum lighting is used to treat neonatal jaundice (bilirubin).

There are other types of Light Therapy that are considered a type of vibrational medicine for use on acupuncture points or meridians, chakras or other areas (see **Gem Therapy**). In these situations specific colors of light are used to stimulate energy centers to improve energy flow. Since light is a type of energy it's believed that different colors have healing effects on the body's energy system.

Standard Light Therapy has been used to treat SAD since the 1980s but is not approved by the FDA due to a shortage of effective testing. If your doctor prescribes Light Therapy your insurance may cover the cost but it is recommended you check with your carrier first. Light boxes may be purchased over-the-counter but it is recommended you discuss treatment with your doctor since there are risks involved including eye damage.

PERCUTANEOUS ELECTRICAL NERVE STIMULATION (PENS) also
Percutaneous Neuromodulation Therapy (PNT)
www.pnthealth.com/files/pntbookletfinal.pdf

A single event of back pain can cause the nerve cells to become hypersensitive, a condition which can continue long after the original injury has healed. In addition to TENS therapy (*see listing*) additional pain relief therapies are **Percuntaneous Electrical Nerve Stimulation** (PENS) and **Percutaneous Neuromodulation Therapy** (PNT). Both are low-risk therapies relying on inserting fine needles through the skin, similar to electrical acupuncture, but placement is not determined by energy meridians as it is with Traditional Chinese Medicine.

For those patients who cannot find back pain relief with TENS therapy these therapies offer additional hope for a non-surgical pain solution. TENS effectiveness can be reduced or eliminated by obesity, scar tissue and other barriers to electrical stimulation. Both PENS and PNT are based on inserting fine-gauge electrodes (about 250 microns in diameter) to a depth of 1 to 4 cm with electrical stimulation of 15 to 30 Hz. PENS placement is located around the painful area so placement is guided by the location of the pain. By comparison PNT therapy places up to 10 electrodes at specific locations in the back. Treatment protocols are for 30-minute sessions up to three times per week for up to ten sessions.

Both types of treatment devices have been approved by the Food and Drug Administration (FDA) for patients suffering from chronic low back or neck pain. In addition there are clinical trials underway at the National Center for Complementary and Alternative Medicine (NCCAM) and the National Institute of Aging (NIA) scheduled for completion in 2007.

PULSED–ELECTROMAGNETIC FIELD THERAPY (PEMF)

www.diapulse.com

Pulsed Electromagnetic Field Therapy (PEMF) is based on the principle that the human body is electrical as well as chemical and that particular frequencies can have healing effects on wounds and disease. The original technology which created negative polarity with electromagnetic waves was developed in the 1930s. One of the earliest research studies was conducted at the Scripps Ranch in 1934 by Milbank Johnson, M.D., Arthur I. Kendall, Ph.D., Professor of Bacteriology at Northwestern University Medical School, E.C. Rosenow Sr., Director of Research at the Mayo Clinic in Rochester, and Royal R. Rife. Their conclusions were that Rife's electromagnetic generator (*also see* **Rife Technology**) either interrupted the reproductive ability of viruses, bacteria and parasites or simply destroyed the pathogens. Tumors were also reported to shrink when exposed to negative polarity.

One machine was developed by Abraham Ginsburg, M.D. and physicist Arthur Milinowski in 1932 but had difficulty becoming accepted until the technology was used successfully to help burns and other wounds heal faster following the Israeli-Arab war in 1967. However in 1972 the FDA stepped in and banned all of the devices, a move that was reversed by a 1987 court order that found the FDA had been "arbitrary and capricious". The technology is currently FDA approved for use for post-operative swelling and pain in soft tissue.

Current models focus electromagnetic energy to a specific body area through a cylindrical treatment head mounted on a moveable arm. The energy easily penetrates clothing, casts, or bandages and has no known side effects.

Because these devices pulse their electromagnetic output, they emit energy for only a fraction of time, allowing any heat associated with the transferred energy to dissipate. Although considered experimental by most insurance companies there are research studies from around the world demonstrating the effectiveness of the principle.

RIFE TECHNOLOGY or Resonant Frequency Therapy
rifehealth.com

Rife Technology, Rife/Bare Device or **Resonant Frequency Therapy** uses a device to produce an electromagnetic wave to put healing energy into the body. The technology is based on the concept that every living entity, including cancer viruses, resonates a unique bio-energy frequency. This device produces specific healing frequencies for each type of illness or disease.

The original device was created by Dr. Royal Raymond Rife in the 1930s to emit energy that would kill a cancer virus inside patients. He was an accomplished scientist and invented the most powerful microscope of its day. There are many stories, almost legends, about its successful medical tests with the Rife Device before it was attacked by the American Medical Association and the California State Medical Society. By 1939 the device had fallen into disfavor and much of the information about the technology was lost for decades.

Today a new version of Resonant Frequency Therapy is available with the Rife/Bare Device which produces four times the amount of electromagnetic energy per watt from improved electronics. Devices may be purchased over the Internet or assembled from do-it-yourself plans.

The list of frequencies for various diseases and illnesses has also improved over the years.

The technology is not FDA approved and no medical claims are made by any manufacturer. Currently they claim the devices can only be sold in America for veterinary use, equipment testing and for personal investigation into the effects of frequencies. The FDA is researching the technology for food safety since it kills pathogens without harming tissue. You can also learn more about Rife Technology by joining one of the Internet user groups like Yahoo's "Rife" group.

USER COMMENTS: *"I have had chronic euticaria on my forearms for the past five years. I have been prescribed medicines which are usually steroids and actizinone cream or phisoderm type products. This usually helps the symptoms of itching and pustules, temporarily at least. My arms are full of pockmark scars from the pustules and blisters that have come and gone over the past years.*

"I ran the device for approx 20 minutes. My arms did not itch for three more days and the pustules started to recede. After the third day I used a euticaria

frequency from another database. All the pustules are gone and healed and I haven't experienced anymore itching or pain.

"I am so happy that something finally worked. Even the dermatologist could not figure out what was causing the condition. But after all methods of treatment failed, yours cured me. Thank you for making the technology available to those of us out here that really need and appreciate your efforts on our behalf."

"She was diagnosed with non-Hodgkin's lymphoma several years ago with obvious tumors in the lymph nodes. The tumors were slow growing, and the expected time of her death was 4-5 years in the future. Suggested treatment consisted of natural supplements to support the immune system and digestion with specific radionics charges for her conditions.

"Within a couple months, there was obvious improvement in all areas. At this writing, she reports that she is free of tumors. This has been confirmed by her MD."

TENS (Transcutaneous Electrical Nerve Stimulator)
www.emedicine.com/pmr/topic206.htm

TENS or **Transcutaneous Electrical Nerve Stimulator** is a pocket-sized electronic device that produces electrical signals to stimulate nerves through the skin for pain relief, typically for the back. A typical unit is battery powered with controls for frequency and intensity, a pulse generator and transformer. The unit is connected by wires to electrodes which stick on the skin.

The TENS unit controls pain by sending electrical signals to the nerves blocking the pain signal to the brain. The positioning of the electrodes on the skin determines which muscles and nerves are stimulated. TENS may also work by stimulating the body's own endorphins in the brain which act to reduce pain.

Electrical stimulation for pain control actually goes back to ancient Greece. Early devices were developed back to the 16th century. Even Benjamin Franklin was a proponent of electricity for pain relief. Dr. C. Norman Shealy created a device called the dorsal column stimulator which contributed to the development of the TENS system. The modern, wearable TENS was patented in 1974 and was originally used for testing patient tolerance to electrical stimulation before a device was implanted in their spinal cord. Many of the patients got so much relief from the TENS unit that they never had the surgery.

The device is available from doctors, physical therapists, chiropractors and over the Internet. While it's possible to use a TENS unit for do-it-yourself experimentation it's beneficial to be trained in the best use of the device by an experienced professional.

USER COMMENTS: *"My chiropractor suggested I try a TENS during a particularly bad episode of lower back pain caused by bulging disks. This wasn't simply a backache but a down-on-your-hands-and-knees situation. I'd* *had back problems for years but this was one of the worst ones and I had a trade show coming up that was vital to my career.*

"The idea of standing on concrete for several hours every day was almost enough to make me break out in a cold sweat. Anyway, my chiropractor showed me how the device works and demonstrated the best place to put the sticky electrodes on my back for my problem. We tested the power and intensity and I wore it for several hours to get used to the sensation.

"You can't imagine the relief that being zapped by electricity can be. It may sound painful but the little irritation of the low-powered TENS unit is nothing compared to the muscle and nerve pain of a bad back. I had to vary the intensity so my back didn't get too used to the sensation and begin to ignore it, but it worked wonderfully. By stimulating the muscles which had almost spasmed into concrete I was able to maintain enough flexibility to move around and function. What an incredible device! Wish I'd learned about it years ago."

BODY CATEGORY SUMMARY

Have you enjoyed the first category of complementary and alternative therapies? Did you discover lots of incredible new possibilities or at least learn more about treatments you've already heard about? Are you beginning to see how the pieces of the puzzle begin to fit together? Can you can see how specific processes fit into general health systems?

The information in this chapter ran the gamut of human history from thousands of years ago (Ayurveda) to the newest inventions (Cold Laser and Pulsed Electromagnetic Field Therapy). You've seen therapies that deal with the entire body like Tai Chi and Rolfing to those that focus on specific problems like Lymph Drainage and Colonic Hydrotherapy. Each one may be just one piece in your puzzle of health.

The Body category could be compared to the rock band you may have played in when you were a teenager. For the most part these techniques are easy to understand, sort of like the four-chord music popular back in the 1960s. You could feel the thumping bass and pounding drumbeat of the music and it's also easy to feel the effects of these body techniques. They may be simple but they can be wonderfully satisfying too.

Chapter 3 – Working with the Mind

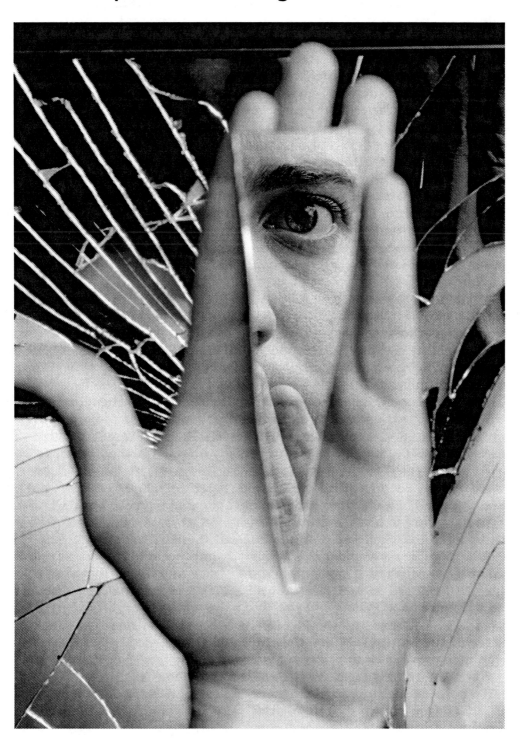

INTRODUCTION TO THE MIND CATEGORY

Many health problems are really problems of emotions, experience or subconscious beliefs seeking physical relief. One doctor is often quoted as saying that up to 80% of the health problems of his patients are really emotional issues. You may already be familiar with people like Louise L. Hay and her book *Heal Your Body* or Narayan Singh Khalsa and his book *Messages From The Body*. The idea of physical problems coming from emotional or psychological causes is not new.

Using the mirror analogy again I could say this might be absent-mindedly placing the mirror on the edge of the counter so it inevitably falls off and breaks. Or it could be a powerful emotional reaction to seeing yourself in the mirror so that you fling it across the room, only to regret doing so the moment it leaves your hand. Or your subconscious could direct your hand to place something heavy on to the mirror to break it. Your mind, conscious and subconscious, influences your behavior and your body in endless ways. The good news is there are new ways to take control of your mind to improve your life and your health.

I'd like to give you an example of this from my life. For years I suffered from painful digestive problems which made my life miserable. As I was going from specialist to specialist in Dallas my condition continued to deteriorate even though my diet has been reduced and simplified until it was about one step short of living on baby food. Eventually I ended up at The Mayo Clinic in Rochester, Minnesota.

Now let me say first of all that I think Mayo is without question the finest medical facility in the world. Their skill and professionalism is second to none and their reputation for excellence is deserved. They did come up with an accurate diagnosis of my problems, something no one else had done, so I will always be indebted to them for their help. However, after days of testing I walked into my doctor's office and he said "I've got good news and I've got bad news. The good news is, your problem isn't going to kill you. The bad news is you're not going to like it and there's very little we can do about it." I was waiting for a drum roll and a punch line but there wasn't one.

As with so many medical conditions I'd simply run into a brick wall with mainstream medicine. They simply didn't have any answers. Being a little stubborn I refused to just give up and suffer and fortunately I discovered Bruce Lipton's book *Biology of Belief* just a few weeks later. From Bruce I discovered Rob Williams and the **PSYCH-K**® process. One class led to another, one technique was added upon the other and slowly, step by step, my health began to improve. A couple of years later my diet is healthier than it's probably ever been and my digestive system is almost normal.

The point of the story is that even when finest doctors don't have a solution, that doesn't mean that there aren't any answers. As you're discovering there are many options available that may be exactly what you need to enjoy a vibrant and healthy life. In my case the problem was a mind-body situation caused by stress and by working on the mind, the body was able to heal.

You're about to discover some amazing techniques in this section. You may have already heard of some of these options like **Animal Assisted Therapy** or **Music Therapy**. There will be some processes or processes that are new to you. So fasten your seat belt and enjoy the ride through the Mind portion of learning how to *UnBreak Your Health*™!

ANIMAL ASSISTED THERAPY
www.deltasociety.org, www.tdi-dog.org

Animal Therapy, or **Animal-Assisted Therapy**, covers a wide range of animals, activities and benefits. Animals are good for the health and well-being of people in a variety of ways. Therapy dogs are familiar to many people but many other types of animals have found helping humans a rewarding pastime including cats, fish, horses and dolphins.

Animal therapy programs are becoming popular in a range of situations including retirement and nursing homes, hospitals, rehabilitation and psychiatric centers, even correctional facilities. Research shows that animals can be beneficial for people in many ways. For example, tanks of tropical fish have helped Alzheimer's patients improve eating habits and reduce disruptive behavior. Riding horses can help improve the balance, coordination and strength of physically challenged individuals. Dolphins can help autistic or disturbed children.

Probably the most common type of animal therapy is done with trained therapy dogs visiting seniors in nursing homes and children in hospitals. Dog owners and their pets go through special training to become qualified for this volunteer effort. The first benefit of a visit from a therapy dog is physical since the petting, reaching and stretching involved is exercise seniors might not experience otherwise. In addition their blood pressure drops and their mental functioning and outlook improves. As pet owners already know, having a friend with a wagging tail around just makes you feel better. Children relax and calm down with a dog around.

Dolphin therapy began in the 1970s in South Florida as a motivation to reinforce selected behaviors in children with Down Syndrome. Today many marine parks offer dolphin therapy for a variety of benefits to people of all ages. There are some reports of dolphins helping to heal health problems, possibly by using their sonar in some way we don't understand yet. Research in this area is at the earliest stage.

If you'd like to learn more about this type of therapy the *Animal-Assisted Therapy and Activities, 9th Ed.* by Phil Arkow is one of the best publications available.

The Delta Foundation was created in 1977 to focus on research in this field. In recent years their mission has built on that scientific and educational base to offer services, including the "Standards of Practice in Animal Assisted Activities and Animal-Assisted Therapy."

Therapy Dogs International was founded in 1976 by a nurse working in England who noticed the benefits of pets interacting with patients. Elaine Smith returned to the U.S. and now operates her organization from California to help bring pet therapy to healthcare facilities.

In case you thought this section might be about complementary and alternative therapies for animals here's a website for the International Alliance for Animal Therapy and Healing at www.iaath.com. As with people, care for animals is becoming more holistic too.

USER COMMENTS: *"I was visiting the West Valley Children's Crisis nursery weekly with my dog. With my history, I really wanted to give back to kids, of any size and age, what ever I could and also do something fun with my furry friend. I'd heard such incredible stories about the impact the teams had made with some of the children.*

"Some of the kids were welcoming, some not interested at all. But I would just 'suit up' and go each week, hoping we could make a difference with just one child. One little boy about 3 or so was so fearful when we would come into the house that he would climb up into the caretaker's arms and begin to cry. He was a little Hispanic boy and I couldn't talk with him much. If we came with in 5 feet of him he would panic and climb up on the back of the couch, we'd just keep assuring him, in calm soft voices that 'it was ok'. After about 3 or 4 visits we were outside on the play ground and lots of kids were running around and playing and stopping by to see us and then run off. I turned around and much to our amazement this little boy had the end of her leash and was following her. At first if she turned around he would drop the leash right away. I'm sure he thought he was walking her like the other kids had done (in fact she was walking him, but it did not matter).

"Later one of the other children wanted to walk her and he said 'NO Mine Dog!'—my heart just melted. On later visits he would see us coming on to the yard and run towards us saying 'Mine Dog' and she would run to him. So I did make a difference in at least one child."

ART THERAPY

www.arttherapy.org

Man has always enjoyed and appreciated the healing power of art. The ability to express emotions visually is recognized as an effective catalyst for personal growth and development. Many consider **Art Therapy** a direct development of Anthroposophically Extended Medicine but it wasn't seen as a separate profession in this country until the 1940s.

Educators have long known that children's art demonstrates their emotional and cognitive growth but psychiatrists began using artwork created by their patients as part of their healing process early in the last century. The creative process of art can enhance recovery and contribute to health and wellness.

Art therapists are professionals trained in both art and therapy. The regulation of art therapists varies by state so please check the situation in your area when looking for an art therapist. In many areas they can become licensed as counselors or mental health therapists. The American Art Therapy Association was founded in 1969 and is the professional organization for this field while the separate Art Therapy Credentials Board certifies the education and experience of therapists.

COGNITIVE BEHAVIORAL THERAPY (CBT)
www.nacbt.org/whatiscbt.htm

Cognitive Behavioral Therapy (CBT) is a type of psychotherapy built on the principle that changing the way a person thinks will also change their behavior and how they feel. The client is an active participant in the correction process for faulty learning experiences and distorted thinking. By recognizing and then correcting negative thoughts and dysfunctional attitudes a new, more positive and productive perspective can reshape their life.

The process begins with a full medical/treatment history of problem. Next a detailed record is made by the patient of each episode so that common factors can be identified. Once a clear picture of the problem or condition is obtained the patient is then given techniques to better ground themselves so they can feel more in control of their situation. These normally include various types of relaxation techniques. The next step in the process is Cognitive Restructuring or learning what thoughts trigger the problem so new, more positive thoughts can take their place.

While normally considered a type of therapy used by trained psychotherapists there are also self-help CBT options available. *FEELING GOOD: The New Mood Therapy* by David D. Burns and Aaron T. Beck was first published in 1980 and it's a wonderful primer on identifying and correcting the distorted thinking involved in depression. They were among the first to say the history of a problem wasn't as important to the patient as changing it in the here and now which began a revolution in traditional talk therapy. It is often considered an alternative type of therapy even today. Research studies are underway involving CBT for several conditions.

The Beck Depression Inventory (BDI, BDI-II) is a twenty-one question test created by Dr. Aaron T. Beck to measure the severity of depression. The first version was published in 1961, revised in 1971 and the BDI-II was published in 1996. It is considered a standard evaluation tool for many situations.

USER COMMENTS: *"If you've ever gone through a carnival Fun House then you know a little about depression. When the world looks upside down and crazy then your feelings and attitudes make perfect sense, at least to you. Reading FEELING GOOD was an eye-opening experience because for the first time I began to recognize all of my stupid thinking errors and began to under-*

stand how they influenced my behavior. Learning to catch my old habits and change them wasn't easy but it has made an incredible difference in my life."

EMDR (Eye Movement Desensitization and Reprocessing)
www.emdr.com, www.emdria.org

EMDR barely qualifies as "alternative therapy" today due to its proven effectiveness and wide acceptance by established medicine, but it is still new enough to be considered outside the mainstream by some. Francine Shapiro discovered in 1987 that eye movements appeared to decrease the negative emotions connected with distressing memories. Eye movements alone did not create a comprehensive therapeutic effect so she added other treatment elements and developed a standard procedure called Eye Movement Desensitization, changing the name in 1991 as a result of further development.

EMDR is an information processing therapy that integrates elements of several different psychotherapies for maximum effect. These include psychodynamic, cognitive behavioral, interpersonal, experiential, and body-centered therapies which are used in an eight-phase sequence. The process uses standardized procedures that include having the client remember difficult or traumatic experiences while simultaneously focusing on an external stimulus such as following the therapist's fingers back and forth with their eyes for 20 or 30 seconds. Therapists also use sounds, tapping or other touch stimulation in this therapy.

Research studies have shown the process very effective in treating traumatic disorders, even Post Traumatic Stress Disorder (PTSD). In 2004 the American Psychiatric Association gave their highest level of recommendation to EMDR for the treatment of trauma. That same year the Department of Veterans Affairs classified EMDR as "strongly recommended."

Training is intended only for licensed or qualified mental health professionals such as graduate students under the supervision of a licensed professional. In the U.S. the EMDR Institute offers training, Francine Shapiro, Ph.D. is the Executive Director. Certification is done by the EMDR International Association (EMDRIA).

USER COMMENTS: *"I was admitted to hospital because of a suicide attempt stemming from a deep depression after 11 years of intense, traditional psychotherapy. My therapist was suggesting I go on full disability because I could not maintain a job. I am young, have a college degree and did not want to live everyday with no purpose to wake up everyday.*

"In the hospital, I was surrounded by many caring, professional healthcare workers including a therapist who practiced EMDR. This was a foreign concept to me, but at that point I was willing to do anything. Since EMDR treatment, I have not had another episode of disassociation. When I came out of the hospital, I did not really believe it was a permanent fix and felt very shaky about getting back into the normality of life but miraculously I have not even had a

close encounter of any kind in 21 months. I am finally starting to believe my healing is permanent.

"I don't care what anyone says, this treatment option is real and it works! I cannot begin to tell you how many medications and therapies I have gone through in the last 11 years to maintain some level of normalcy in my life. I wanted to get better and did anything anyone suggested but nothing seemed to work fully. I really hate that I was at the end of my rope when I accidentally discovered EMDR therapy, but I am forever thankful to the EMDR therapist and the time she took to help me."

EXPRESSIVE WRITING also Journaling

www.writingtoheal.com/

Expressive Writing is a personal essay about your deepest thoughts, feelings and stressful events in your life. Also known as the writing cure it can be a form of journaling for self-awareness and therapy or can be part of a classroom situation. It allows writers to express themselves about problems in their life which frequently produces beneficial results. It's also called **Journaling**.

Although the technique has been used since the beginning of writing, one of the earliest reported studies was in 1983 by psychologist James Pennebaker. Research continues to show that writing deep thoughts and feelings provides beneficial stress release which improves the writer's outlook. Expressive writing has also been shown to boost the writer's immune system, improve grades, decrease blood pressure and reduce pain. Studies are currently underway in several areas including at National Center for Complimentary and Alternative Medicine (NCCAM), a division of the National Institutes of Health.

General recommendations are to write at a quiet time of day when you can concentrate for at least 15 or 20 minutes and write non-stop without worrying about spelling or grammar. Write for at least three or four days in a row, it doesn't matter if you write about the same subject or change the focus of your writing frequently. If writing about painful events makes you sad or depressed, like seeing a sad movie, the effect should go away after a few hours. However if it persists, the best suggestion is to simply stop writing or change topics.

The technique is also used by many professional therapists in the course of therapy.

There are several books on the subject including *The Writing Cure: How Expressive Writing Promotes Health and Emotional Well-Being* by Stephen J. Lepore and Joshua M. Smyth.

USER COMMENTS: *"I felt that the (expressive writing) helped me greatly deal with the problems at hand. It's one thing for you to tell yourself something or for you to get advice from an outside source, but for me to see the writing on* *the page that MY hand was creating and to read the thoughts that were flowing from MY head...it kind of put everything into perspective."*

"I felt it had a very positive effect because it was the first time that many of these thoughts were made 'tangible' and it felt good to get them out. I had neither written nor talked about these feelings before to anyone, and getting them out on paper helped me sort out my feelings."

"Although I have not talked with anyone about what I wrote, I was finally able to deal with it, work through the pain instead of trying to block it out. Now it doesn't hurt to think about it."

"Putting the painful things on paper and reading them over and over made me realize that they can no longer hurt me. That was better than the years of therapy that I have had."

FORGIVENESS THERAPY (FT) also Radical Forgiveness
www.forgiving.org, www.radicalforgiveness.com

Forgiveness Therapy empowers a person to forgive in order for them to heal. Claire Frazier-Yzaguirre wrote: *"When we forgive, we free ourselves from the bitter ties that bind us to the one who hurt us."* Forgiveness is something we all would like to see in the world. A frequently quoted poll says that while 94% of Americans think it's important to forgive, only 48% said they usually tried to forgive others. While we want to forgive it can be a struggle between two conflicting energies within; the need to condemn versus the desire to forgive. While revenge may be sweet we pay a high price for it by staying a victim. With forgiveness we discover self-empowerment, better health, more energy, better relationships and many other benefits.

Research at the University of Wisconsin in 1997 demonstrated that forgiveness could be taught with positive results. It's been shown to be especially beneficial in the treatment of addictions. Many therapists and medical professionals have been trained in Forgiveness Therapy to help patients appreciate the benefits of forgiveness. There are also self-help books available.

One of the most vivid examples of forgiveness was Pope John Paul II's meeting with his would-be assassin, Mehmet Ali Agca. While most religions of the world advocate forgiveness this was leadership by example of the highest order.

Radical Forgiveness is a different paradigm presented by Colin C. Tipping in his book *Radical Forgiveness: Making Room for the Miracle*. This process uses spiritual intelligence, that part of your awareness which understands it isn't about struggle, but attracting what you want from the sea of abundance known as the universe. By using the spiritual technology of Radical Forgiveness we raise our vibration level and heal the past.

The core belief of Radical Forgiveness is that everything happens for a reason, there are no mistakes and there are no victims. This spiritual perspective believes that every situation is divinely guided and happened not to us, but for us, because it was meant to happen for the highest good of all concerned. In fact, our Higher Selves created the experience for our healing and spiritual growth. It is a shift in energy and perspective.

The Institute of Radical Forgiveness offers courses and certification of coaches and facilitators.

USER COMMENTS: *"Over the years, I sincerely thought I had forgiven my ex-husband. Radical Forgiveness taught me that I hadn't. Not only that, but that I was still carrying baggage around. After Radical Forgiveness, I immediately felt different towards my ex-husband and have continued to feel so ever since. It is as though some unseen cord has somehow been cut, and I am finally free."*

"Radical Forgiveness is the most effective tool for writing your own ticket out of 'victimland.' It embraces the physical, spiritual, emotional, developmental and intellectual realms to see the beauty and perfection of the life you have, and propels you toward authentic and lasting change. The beauty of Radical Forgiveness is in its simplicity and EVERYONE stands to benefit and grow from this valuable experience."

"I have spent the past 45 years dealing with the death of my mother when I was eight years old. My entire life has been a deep and unfilled hole. Fortunately, the workshop was a miracle for me and my life changed. I am so at peace and so fulfilled in my life. It was my miracle. I now have great inner prosperity, my life is rich with true abundance. I have a loving and fulfilled relationship with myself, and my inner self is tranquil. I have just succeeded at two philanthropic projects … I could not imagine achieving more than I feel today. I will always love you for giving me my life. My true, joyous life."

GUIDED IMAGERY

www.AcademyForGuidedImagery.com,

www.GuidedImageryInc.com/guided.html

We all were using imagery before we learned to speak because it's how the subconscious mind learns and remembers - through the senses. The most powerful part of our brain uses sights, sounds, smells, tastes and touch. That's the reason your memories all come back to you as collections of sensory information instead of words describing the memory. It's also the way the mind communicates with the body. **Guided Imagery** uses the power of our subconscious and imagination to produce positive mind/body responses.

Imagery has been used all over the world for thousands of years; it's a vital part of many religions such as Hinduism and Judaism. It's been used by such diverse cultures as the ancient Greeks and Egyptians to the Navaho Indians of America. Today visualizations are used by athletes who perform better when they see, feel and experience their sport before they actually do it. It's recommended by experts from Dale Carnegie to Robert Schuller to Steven Covey to produce peak performances.

Estimates are that at least half of the thousands of thoughts we have every day are negative. This steady stream of negative images produces stress which can alter your body, making you more susceptible to a variety of illnesses. Learning to direct and control the images in your head can help your body heal itself. It's especially effective for treatment of stress-related conditions and is used as a part of various relaxation techniques.

Recommendations on Guided Imagery are to invest 15 to 20 minutes each day along with a relaxation technique. It may take time to master but patience and persistence are the key factors to success. Simply loosen any restrictive clothing, take off shoes and sit comfortably in a chair. You may want to dim the lights. Close your eyes and begin to breathe deeply in a slow, measured manner. It may be beneficial to picture yourself descending an imaginary staircase to help deepen the relaxation.

When you're feeling very relaxed you can imagine a favorite place or enjoyable moment with family or friends. Try to imagine the same scene each time your practice because it will create a safe place where you'll feel secure and become more receptive to other images. Once you're comfortable you can begin to move your attention towards your ailment or problem. If several images come to mind just choose one and focus on it for that session. If no images come to mind try focusing on a different sensation or think about your feelings at that moment.

Another technique is called "**painting**" and you simply close your eyes and concentrate on the color black to create a canvas. When you've managed to color the entire field of vision in your mind you can then begin to mentally replace it with a color you associate with tension or your problem. Then simply replace that color with one that you find relaxing, like changing from a bright red to a soft blue. You can also replace it with a relaxing scene like walking on the beach or watching the sunset.

There are many techniques to guide the images and sensory information in your mind. In health situations patients are frequently urged to picture their organs and body systems functioning perfectly, tumors can be seen shrinking or immune cells conquering microorganisms. Guided Imagery can also be used with affirmations which are most effective when positive and present-tense.

There are many self-help books, CD's, training classes and videos available from different schools of guided imagery. While many medical professionals have been trained in these techniques it's also possible to find help from various types of coaches and complimentary or alternative healing practitioners. The process is beginning to find its way into fitness and health clubs across the country for stress relief. It is recommended that you research the training and qualifications of any care provider for Guided Imagery.

The 2002 federal survey of complementary and alternative medicine found that 3.0% of those surveyed had experienced guided imagery and 2.1% of those surveyed had experienced it in the previous year.

The Academy for Guided Imagery was established in 1989 to set professional standards and certification in its specialty, **Interactive Guided Imagery**sm but there are also other organizations that offer specialized training such as **Beyond Ordinary Nursing**.

USER COMMENTS: *"I can't believe what a difference (guided imagery) made in my pre- and post (heart valve surgery) stress and pain. Thank you … for caring for me, the patient, as a whole and not just a number."*

"My doctor encouraged me to listen to … guided imagery … before, during and after major cancer surgery. It's been eight years and I still listen to it to cope with personal and professional issues."

"In addition to providing this option to our patients we have found that our staff, in particular our nursing staff, have come to appreciate this tool for self use."

HUMOR
www.aath.org, www.cancerclub.com, www.rxlaughter.org

It's often been said by those outside the mainstream medical community that "laughter may indeed be the best medicine", possibly because it's affordable but also because it's true. **Humor Therapy** is often considered a type of Psychoneuroimmunology (*see listing*) but this subject deserves its own listing. Everyone already knows how laughter makes you feel good and full of joy, but I put so much importance on this subject because I've enjoyed the movie *Patch Adams* starring Robin Williams too much!

Doctors didn't seriously consider laughter a legitimate form of therapy until the New England Journal of Medicine published the Norman Cousins case study in 1979 showing how laughter could reverse a serious disease. Norman Cousins published *Anatomy of an Illness* in 1964 about his fight with ankylosing spondylitis, a painful disintegration of the connective tissue in the spine. He designed his own humor therapy and discovered that 15 minutes of laughter could bring him up to two hours of pain-free sleep. Since that time laughter has been found to lower blood pressure, reduce stress hormones, boost immune system function and release endorphins, the body's natural pain killers. A good belly laugh is considered a type of exercise providing good cardiac conditioning for those unable to perform regular physical exercise. Best of all, it produces a wonderful sense of well being. It's also a great coping mechanism and is increasingly used for the treatment of cancer.

Today doctors are often still afraid to use humor. There is no reference to humor therapy in most medical training manuals or programs. There has been very little research because humor can't be patented and no research means there are no articles in professional journals. Doctors may also be concerned that it may reduce the professional distance from the patient. All of these are "old school" problems that are slowly fading away as the overwhelming benefits of humor become more accepted.

One example is the Big Apple Circus in New York which created Clown Care twenty years ago to entertain children. Today they have 84 professional clowns working at hospitals in cities across the country. New York-Presbyterian Hospital has these clowns working at the Morgan Stanley Children's Hospital three days each week all year long.

Over a decade ago a doctor in India, Dr. Madan Kataria, created Laughter Yoga as a result of his research on laughter. Today there are thousands of Laughter Clubs and other groups around the world to spread the benefits of laughter. One of the most important benefits of laughter is that you live in the moment. Focusing on the beauty of life right now has many wonderful effects.

The Association for Applied and Therapeutic Humor (AATH) was created in 1987 to "advance the understanding and application of humor and laughter for their positive benefits". It is an international community of professionals who incorporate humor into their daily lives.

USER COMMENTS: *(From a hospital clown) "I went to see a boy with cancer who was about to lose his leg. He asked if there was any way to avoid it and I had to answer him 'No' but then I asked him what he'd like to do. He said 'Jump on the bed'. So I climbed up on to his hospital bed and we both jumped up and down right up to the time when they came to take him to surgery. I gave him something to take with him so he'd see it when he first woke up to bring a smile to his face."*

"I really love creating a welcoming atmosphere for kids in the hospital because it also helps the parents remember the child and not the illness. We have to react to each child differently when we ask to enter the room. If they're quiet then we respond in a quiet manner. Sometimes they're angry so we help them release it at the clown or in a comedic manner like a paper-towel duel. Finding laughter in the worst of circumstances isn't easy but it is so rewarding."

(From a doctor) "Bringing joy, laughter and play calls them to their natural state of health."

"I first learned about humor therapy from a dear friend dying with cancer. She watched every funny movie or show ever made, over and over, because it relieved her pain and gave her a feeling of happiness for a few moments. Ever since then I start each day by reading the funnies first to begin the day with a chuckle. I take my wife to see almost every animated movie and comedy we can find. I'm determined not to wait until I'm dying to see the beauty and humor in every day."

HYPNOSIS
www.asch.net, en.wikipedia.org/wiki/Hypnosis

Hypnosis is called a state of mind where communication with the subconscious mind is enabled while bypassing the conscious mind. While there is general agreement about some of the effects of hypnosis, there are a variety of definitions of hypnosis and many different theories about how and why it works. If you've ever driven several miles and not known how you got there you've experienced a type of hypnosis called highway hypnosis. It's a similar sensation to reading a book intently or focusing completely on a TV program so that you become unaware of your surroundings.

There are three major styles of hypnosis are: Suggestion; Mental Imagery and Self. The first type is where a trained hypnotist speaks softly and rhythmically to produce an enhanced state of relaxation. With the second style the hypnotist talks about specific scenes to produce focused concentration. The third type is self-explanatory.

Hypnotherapy or clinical hypnosis is often used to treat conditions such as phobias, anxiety and chronic pain. It's also used for age regression therapy, enhancing self-esteem and improving memory and concentration. It's been used in medicine for anesthesia and for childbirth along with other conditions. Hypnosis is even used by dentists to control fear, saliva and gagging. Lay hypnotists use it to help clients stop smoking, to lose weight and to activate the mind-body connection to aid in the treatment of fibromyalgia, cancer, diabetes, and arthritis.

Franz Anton Mesmer, a charismatic healer, developed the forerunner of hypnosis in the 18th century. Surgeon James Braid coined the term hypnosis in 1843 referring to Hypnos, the Greek god of sleep because of the resemblance of mesmerism to sleep. Modern hypnosis is due to pioneers like Clark Hull and his student Milton Erikson. Eriksonian Hypnosis uses a passive technique to work with the subconscious instead of the regular commanding style. The American Medical Association approved the use of hypnosis in 1958 and the American Psychological Association accepted it in 1960.

Many people confuse stage hypnotism with hypnotherapy, failing to appreciate that stage hypnotists screen their volunteers to select the most cooperative, possibly with exhibitionist tendencies. This type of entertainment perpetuates a myth about hypnosis which discourages people from seeking legitimate hypnotherapy.

According to the 2002 federal survey of CAM use in America 1.8% reported they had experienced hypnosis at some time and 0.2% had used it in the prior 12 months.

There is no accredited qualification to practice hypnosis and in the U.S. so certified lay hypnotists can perform "non-therapeutic hypnotism" instead of hypnotherapy. There are laws in 16 states which regulate the practice of hypnotism: California; Connecticut; Colorado; Florida; Idaho; Illinois; Indiana; Minnesota; New Jersey; New Hampshire; New Mexico; North Carolina; Rhode Island; and Utah. There are changes happening in 2007 in Connecticut, New York and Minnesota. Washington and Nevada have statutes for forensic hypnosis only. Please check with your state regarding current regulations and requirements. The American Society of Clinical Hypnosis and the Society for Clinical and Experimental Hypnosis are the only nationally recognized organizations for licensed healthcare professionals using hypnosis so you can use their websites to locate professionals in your area.

USER COMMENTS: *"Like a lot of folks I went to a hypnotist to help me quit the 2-packs-a-day smoking habit I'd had for more than fifteen years. It was a relaxing process. The hypnotist began the session by having me close my eyes and relax. We went to safe, relaxing places and counted the steps down to deeper relaxation. I never felt any loss of control or awareness, just openness to new and better ideas.*

I think the self-help tape he gave me to use as needed was an important factor in my finally being able to quit after many, many attempts. Going to sleep listening to the tape reinforced my desire not to smoke and seemed to give me more willpower to resist the urges."

MEDITATION

www.meditationsociety.com,   www.relaxationresponse.org

The term **Meditation** has different meanings to different people. It's used to describe a wide range of practices with many different goals but we generally associate the term with turning our attention inward. It is used most often to relieve stress and provide a feeling of peace. It also can be used for personal or spiritual development and for healing.

Meditation comes from a variety of Eastern traditions and there are a variety of techniques involved in meditation depending on the spiritual tradition and/or practitioner. Meditation can involve focusing on a specific object, on the background or shifting between the two. Postures may be sitting, lying down, kneeling or being cross-legged. In almost every case the spine should be kept straight for proper energy flow. Time requirements also vary widely but generally 20-30 minutes per day is accepted as a normal amount of time for meditation.

Transcendental Meditation® (TM) is one of the most recognized forms of meditation. This is the program of Maharishi Mahesh Yogi which promotes two twenty-minute sessions of meditation each day in a seated position with eyes closed. Training involves the awarding of a unique mantra for each individual to fully experience the restful alertness. Most of the research on the health effects of meditation has been done on TM.

Another style of meditation is called the **Relaxation Response** after the eponymous book (1995) by Herbert Benson, M.D. and Associate Professor of Medicine at the Harvard Medical School. Separating the beneficial effects of meditation from religious connotations, Dr. Benson's research showed that repetition of a sound, word, phrase or even movement and simply putting intruding thoughts aside could create the Relaxation Response. This was the counter to our stress response, also called the fight-or-flight response.

While it may be difficult to image any negative effects from meditation there are reports of problems, especially if it's practiced incorrectly or too intensely. Credible teachers of meditation will warn students about potential problems.

According to the recent federal research on the use of complementary and alternative medicine 10.2% of Americans reported they'd used meditation at some time and 7.6% said they'd used it in the prior year.

MINDFULNESS

en.wikipedia.org/wiki/Mindfulness or
www.budsas.org/ebud/mfneng/mind0.htm

Mindfulness is becoming intentionally aware of your thoughts and actions in the present moment in a totally non-judgmental manner. It is also an approach to life based on being fully awake in our lives to access our own inner resources for healing and insight. Mindfulness has been around for thousands of years and is a fundamental part of Buddhism but today Western therapists are also embracing it as an effective way to deal with depression and anxiety.

Mindfulness is simply being aware of your present moment without judging or thinking, you simply are "in the moment". It's been said that a moment is like a breath because both are replaced by the next one. An ancient Japanese saying explains it as: "Wherever you go, there you are." Mindfulness is a way to accept that the past is history and nothing can change it, while the future is not here yet, so there is no need to worry about it. Being "in the moment" helps us to appreciate that the gift of life is right now.

Mindfulness does not have to be limited to a formal meditation session, it can be done at any time in almost any way because it is simply bringing the mind into focus on the present moment. If you're walking and notice the feel of the ground underneath your feet, the wind on your face and everything going on around you, you're practicing a type of mindfulness.

A more formal style of Mindfulness in meditation is to give a label to each breath in and out to help concentrate attention on the moment and to disregard the mind's usual running commentary. Mindfulness can bring about an awareness that happiness isn't brought about by a change in your external situation, it originates inside.

There are two different types of mindful meditation in Buddhism called Vipassana and Samatha. Vipassana is translated as "insight" or the full awareness of what is happening as it happens. Samatha is considered "concentration" or tranquility, that state when the mind is brought to rest and not allowed to wander. Most systems of meditation focus on Samatha and use a prayer, candle or other device to exclude all other thoughts.

Mindfulness is the basic component of **Mindfulness Based Stress Reduction** (*see listing*) and **Mindfulness Based Cognitive Therapy** (*see listing*). One of the leading centers of research and practice of mindfulness is at the University of Massachusetts Center for Mindfulness in Medicine, Healthcare, and Society.

MINDFULNESS BASED COGNITIVE THERAPY (MBCT)

www.mbct.co.uk

Mindfulness Based Cognitive Therapy is a combination of Cognitive Behavior Therapy (*see listing*) with Mindfulness (*see listing*) meditation techniques developed by Zindel Segal, Mark Williams and John Teasdale in 2002. The technique is based on Jon Kabat-Zinn's Mindfulness Based Stress Reduction program (*see listing*) created in 1979. In 2001, Bruno Cayoun developed a 4-stage model with the same name but later changed the name to **Mindfulness-Integrated Cognitive Behavior Therapy** (MiCBT) to differentiate the two therapies.

Both MBCT and MiCBT reduce the relapse rate of depression by helping patients recognize and deal with undesired feelings as they appear instead of pushing them away. Patients who've suffered depression have an increased risk of recurrence because it takes less triggering for each subsequent episode.

The MBCT process is taught in 8 weekly classes with tapes and video homework between sessions along with an all-day session about week 6. It teaches yoga stretches and simple breathing meditations to help participants become more aware of the present moment. Education about depression includes cognitive therapy exercises to demonstrate the links between thinking and feelings. Patients learn what makes them susceptible to downward mood spirals, why they become "stuck" at the bottom and how to choose their responses instead of simply reacting automatically. The United Kingdom's *National Institute of Clinical Excellence* (NICE) has endorsed MBCT as an effective treatment for the prevention of depression relapse.

In addition to therapy classes, be sure to look for *The Mindful Way Through Depression* (2007).

MINDFULNESS BASED STRESS REDUCTION (MBSR)

www.umassmed.edu/cfm/srp/index.aspx

Mindfulness Based Stress Reduction is much more than the name implies, it's a process of intentionally focused awareness of the present moment without judgment as a method of self-reflection. MBSR operates without the restrictive attitudes of yourself, others or the world. When Jon Kabat-Zinn, Ph.D. began a new type of alternative health program at the University of Massachusetts Medical School in 1979 he called it the Stress Reduction Clinic because meditation was considered too "far out" to be taken seriously at the time. As news of his results spread throughout the hospital more difficult cases were referred to him and his success continued to grow. The program became more accepted and continued to expand, eventually becoming The Center for Mindfulness in Medicine, Healthcare and Society.

Today the program is a course of 8 weekly classes with one full day of class on a Saturday or Sunday. It includes gentle stretching and mindful Yoga exercises along with guided instruction into methods of mindfulness meditation. There are also exercises to improve awareness of everyday life, group dialogue, individual instruction and daily homework assignments using tapes and workbooks. It's a challenging but life-affirming process as participants learn to relate to what's happening in their lives in a positive new way by learning how to take charge. The process also teaches you how to do what no one else can do for you, consciously and systematically work through your own stress, pain, illness or other life challenge.

MBSR also taps directly into the spiritual discipline of the heart, spirit, soul, Tao, Dharma or other name. This type of present-moment awareness helps you to experience your life not only with acceptance but also an eager curiosity and appreciation. Participants learn to open their eyes to the pleasures of their life and improve their skills for tapping into their own wisdom and internal resources.

There have been decades of research on MBSR since the program's inception documenting the many benefits of the process. Participants increase their ability to relax but also experience decreases in physical problems like pain and psychological symptoms with a corresponding increase in self-esteem, energy and enthusiasm for life.

Today more than 13,000 people have completed the MBSR program and there are more than 300 trained practitioners involved in programs at hundreds of hospitals around the country. The program has been featured in the Bill Moyers' PBS documentary *Healing and the Mind,* on Oprah, NBC's *Dateline*, ABC's *Chronicle* and in other programs and articles. Jon Kabat-Zinn's book *Full Catastrophe Living* provides an introduction to mindfulness training.

MUSIC THERAPY

www.musictherapy.org

Although **Music Therapy** goes back to ancient times the modern concept originated in veterans hospitals after the wars when doctors noticed the beneficial physical and emotional responses to music from visiting musicians. Today it improves the quality of life for children and adults suffering from disabilities or disease by improving motor skills, social and cognitive development and even spiritual awareness. A music therapist frequently uses Music Therapy techniques with broader types of therapy.

Patients do not have to have any musical abilities to benefit from Music Therapy. There isn't one particular type of music that is more beneficial than others. The type of music chosen for therapy will depend on the patient's preferences, situation and type of assistance needed. Listening to music you enjoy will relieve stress but hearing music you dislike can create it. Music can be used to help motor skills develop in children with special needs or adults recovering from stroke. Simply listening to music can help memory function in the elderly. Classical and jazz music are often credited with improving mental functions due to their complex arrangements.

Stress reduction is a popular form of music therapy which does not require a trained therapist. Listening to your favorite music works on many levels to wash away the stress of the day, often called a "sound bath". For best results enjoy at least twenty minutes of slow music with a rhythm of less than 72 beats per minute – the natural heart beat. Concentrate on the silence between the notes to keep your mind from analyzing the music and remember to focus on slow, rhythmic breathing. This type of music therapy can even be combined with exercise when you take your favorite tunes on a walk.

Professional music therapists often are designated by MT-BC (Music Therapist, Board-Certified) or the designation of CMT, ACMT, or RMT. Today the American Music Therapy Association sets the standards for education and clinical training. Music Therapy may be covered by government or private insurance so remember to check with your provider.

USER COMMENTS: *"In my practice I've found that music that's familiar is able to grab the attention of somebody with dementia and engages them in the moment of that experience, so much so that the attention and the holding of that attention allows for other functioning to happen."*

NEURO LINGUISTIC PROGRAMMING (NLP)

www.nlp-world.com, www.nlpinfo.com/

NeuroLinguistic Programming is both a name and its definition because its three basic components are neurology, language and our programming. NLP develops better understanding of the thinking and cognitive awareness behind behaviors based on a constantly evolving process. How we experience life and encode our experiences will affect our behavior and communication so NLP makes it possible to transform our beliefs and grow as individuals, it helps you run your own mind to improve your life. The process is applicable for learning, developing peak performance, in psychotherapy, for business, and personal communication.

NLP has two basic features: The map is not the territory, and Life and Mind are systemic processes. We never really know reality, we only know our perceptions of reality, so we can change our "map" about life since they're only our perceptions, not reality. The second part is that we naturally seek an optimal state of balance in our lives using self-organizing processes. NLP uses a variety of techniques including eye position, body language, communication and awareness.

The initial ideas of NLP were developed by Richard Bandler, John Grinder and Gregory Bateson in 1973. The term describes a set of models and principles about how the mind, neurology and language patterns are involved in our subjective reality and resulting behaviors.

You can experience NLP through books, DVDs, seminars and private practitioners of NLP. The process can be used for self development or to assist others.

USER COMMENTS: *"I took the Diamonds of the Mind course originally. As with many techniques, the more you practice the principles the better you get at them, and the more natural they become. The challenge is to remember to slow down long enough to actually intentionally use what you've learned.*

"I do feel very empowered and wise. Like I have a 'special secret' that I can fall back on, to help me through the difficult challenges in life and help others as well. NLP has allowed me to see life from a different perspective. I've become more tolerant, more accepting, less critical and a better listener. By looking for the good in others and for better ways to communicate, your life becomes richer.

"Another technique I use a lot, and I can't remember the technical name for it, is for when someone is "in your face" being very negative or obnoxious. You simply cut through the air slowly with your hand and draw an imaginary boundary between you and that person or that thought, to separate you from their negative energy. It's great!"

ONE BRAIN™ SYSTEM
www.3in1concepts.net

The **One Brain™ System** is a combination of kinesiology with behavioral genetics created by Gordon Stokes and Daniel Whiteside to integrate the mind, body and spirit. It is a program of self-discovery to remove obstacles from each person, to empower them to fulfill their essential purpose in life.

The process is based on the concept that if we experience negative stress when learning something new then whenever we experience that activity again we also re-experience the negative stress. If we are basing our choices on negative experiences from our past then we are sacrificing our freedom to choose today and become locked into a pattern of limitation and denial. The goal of Three In One is to enhance performance and quality of life by giving people the power to choose.

This process has several features to assess negative stress imbalances and correct them. Their Behavioral Barometer™ identifies where the individual is right now emotionally and where they would like to go in their life. The Emotional Stress Defusion process reduces stress on any issue in the client's life. The System also uses a type of kinesiology called Clear-Circuit Muscle Testing with their Age Regression technique so that all corrections release negative stress factors in both past and present. The process has been used to improve reading and skills, artistic expression, physical coordination and sports performance among other with other types of problems.

Individuals can use the One Brain™ System with a qualified facilitator or they may take the series of classes to learn the skills for themselves.

One Brain™ System is a registered trademark of Three In One.

USER COMMENTS: *"Going through school had been a struggle for me because I had dyslexia and some other learning disabilities. I did graduate, but not without some very deep-seated emotional issues connected to my experiences. When it became clear that I was going to need further education to continue with my future, a lot of anxiety started to rise as well as all my fears from my school days. I found a therapist who did Three In One Concepts, which uses kinesiology to defuse stress from past traumas. This was the best gift I could have ever received, it allowed me to flourish with confidence and strengthen my self-esteem. 'What the mind believes the body perceives', and with kinesiology it helps you to understand what the body is perceiving."*

ORGONE THERAPY

www.orgonomicscience.org

After years of research Austrian psychiatrist and scientist William Reich, M.D. developed Orgone Therapy in the 1930s to treat emotional and physical illness by removing barriers to healthy expressions of emotion and sexual feeling. After studying with Sigmund Freud he created a new approach he described as Character Analysis which concerned characteristic behaviors. Later he added analysis of the physical expression of patient attitudes, a concept he labeled Armor. The combination of these two methods became Orgone Therapy.

Reich believed that all life processes, including our sexuality, are expressions of the biological energy of the body he called orgone energy. To be healthy this energy must be free to pulsate and flow unrestricted by the armor an individual develops to protect themself. He developed a device called an accumulator to collect orgone energy from the atmosphere which he felt was beneficial to living things. The device landed him in court when the FDA challenged his research. Because he refused to defend his work in a courtroom he was found guilty of failing to obey an injunction and jailed. In 1957 he died while still in prison.

Orgone Therapy allows the therapist the flexibility to move between verbal and physical modes as the situation requires with emphasis more on "how" the patient defends rather than on the "why". The biophysical work usually begins the furthest away from the genitals and gradually progresses towards the pelvis and deeper issues. Sessions are normally done once per week but individuals with self-destructive behaviors such as alcohol or drug abuse are not viable candidates for Orgone Therapy.

Orgone therapists are required to have clinical psychotherapy training and be certified in their chosen field of psychotherapy. In addition they must have careful supervision to help them maintain a professional distance and appropriate boundaries. Since 1982 the Institute for Orgonomic Science has promoted Orgone Therapy and its continued research. Today the American College of Orgonomy provides CME approved training in medical orgonomy to qualified physicians.

PSYCH-K®

www.psych-k.com

Originally called **Psychological Kinesiology**, **PSYCH-K**® uses muscle testing to work directly with the subconscious mind. It's called accelerated personal growth by creator Robert M. Williams, M.A., a non-invasive, interactive process for change. Developed in the late 1980s it is based on the formula: Beliefs=Thoughts/Feelings=Actions=Reality. The PSYCH-K® process is a unique method to locate problem subconscious beliefs and quickly transform them into beliefs which support your best life.

The process uses the straight-arm style of muscle testing with light to moderate pressure by the facilitator. The goal is to obtain either a "lock" or "unlock" response to a statement spoken by either the facilitator or client. A locked or straight arm indicates a yes/positive response while a weak or unlocked arm is a no/negative answer.

There are seven major types of balances used to change subconscious beliefs. This technique is done with the client, it's not something that's done to a client. After locating a problem belief and selecting a balance style the facilitator must also receive permission and commitment from the client's subconscious for the work. If the muscle test response is weak or unlocked, the session is finished.

Training and certification is done by the founder or a Certified Instructor. State regulations on facilitators vary depending on whether the process is classified as a massage technique or not so please check with your local agencies.

PSYCH-K® is a registered trademark of The Myrddin Corporation.

USER COMMENTS: *"Muscle testing is weird. You can experience it and still have a hard time believing it. Your arm stays straight and strong when you say 'My name is ____' and that makes sense. It gets weak and falls down when you try to lie and say 'My name is Bugs Bunny.' At first you think it has to be the facilitator changing how much pressure they're using but eventually you accept the fact that they're very consistent and somehow your subconscious is getting into the process.*

"At first the Balances were short and simple. It was hard to tell if anything was really happening. The muscle testing said something had changed but the balance was so subtle it was hard to tell. Then I did a different kind of Balance, sort of a graduation to a higher form, and boy was it different!

"This new balance took a lot of time. Okay, it was only 15 minutes but it felt like hours. As I got close to the end I noticed that tears were running down my cheeks. For a guy, this was very, very strange. It's not like I was remembering any terrible events in my life or thinking disturbing thoughts, but the balance was on a major issue in my life. Clearly something was happening this time! When it was over I felt such a sense of freedom and calm it was wonderful but strange at the same time. So this is what dramatic change feels like. By the

way, in the months following the balance there was substantial improvement in the problem."

"Preparing for a trip to Dominica a client did several Balances on his terrible fear of heights. Afterwards he reported "I rode the Rainforest tram with no problems, only a slight bit of apprehension when we crossed the Breakfast River gorge 300 feet below (which I think was more being anxious that my fear would return than a fear of the height itself). On the return trip, when the tram is actually about 10 feet higher, there was no apprehension and I was able to look over the side at the river below. For bonus points, I usually gain 5-7 lbs on a one week vacation, but this time I lost one pound!"

"One of my clients was nervous when speaking in public, and she was scheduled to do three professional speaking engagements the following week. We did one two-hour session (the first PSYCH-K® session she had ever had). We worked with a goal statement for how she wanted to feel when speaking (relaxed, engaged and enjoying herself), which required a VAK to the Future; after the VAK she tested strong on her goal. Next, a supporting balance was indicated using Belief Points, which we did.

"She just called to report how relaxed she felt during the three speaking engagements, how engaged she felt with the audience, and how she enjoyed it. She said that PSYCH-K® must have made the difference, since she hadn't worked with any other tools to produce the change."

SEDONA METHOD®

www.sedona.com

The **Sedona Method**® is a self-help technique for releasing unwanted feelings and emotions which may be having a negative effect on your life. The process consists of a series of questions to ask yourself which will increase your awareness of the moment and enable you to use your natural ability to let go of those feelings quickly.

The process is based on the concept that we're limited only by the thoughts and feelings we hold in our minds. If you feel powerful you will then act in a powerful manner, just as if you feel sad you will act that way. The Sedona Method® functions on the emotional level and it also affects how you act too, so you can make better decisions and be more in control of your life. It balances both left and right hemispheres of the brain, appealing to men and women.

The process was developed by Lester Levenson in 1952 to save his own life. He'd been sent home to die but instead the 42-year-old physicist and entrepreneur created the Sedona Method® and after using it for three months his health and happiness were restored. The first class in the technique was held in 1974 in Sedona, Arizona.

Hale Dwoskin met Mr. Levenson in 1976 and became the heir to all of the Sedona Method® copyrights so he could continue Mr. Levenson's work. Mr.

Dwoskin was the co-founder in 1996 of Sedona Training Associates and is currently CEO. He is also the author of *The Sedona Method: Your Key To Lasting Happiness, Success, Peace and Emotional Well-Being.*

The Sedona Method can be learned by home-study course or at authorized seminars.

USER COMMENTS: *"I have read before that The Sedona Method could help people with physical problems, but I NEVER in a million years thought that could be true for me. Well, I have had a gnawing, ulcer-type pain for years that left on my second day of releasing at the Seven-Day Retreat. The Method works!"*

"My blood pressure was recorded to be 180/90 previous to my taking the course. Since then, my last blood pressure reading was 140/80 (without taking the prescribed drugs)."

"I had several physical ailments, including migraine headaches, diverticulitis, gout, and severe hypoglycemia, and had imminent surgery scheduled. But within a few days after beginning to release, the surgical condition disappeared and never reappeared. My other physical problems also cleared up."

SHAMANISM

www.shamanism.org/

Shamanism is based on the premise that the visible world is pervaded by invisible forces or spirits that affect the lives of the living. There is archaeological evidence that this practice has existed for more than 20,000 years and on every continent which means it predates all organized religions.

While there are shamanistic practices unique to each culture there are some common, if not quite universal, features. A shaman is usually an intermediary traveling between the real world and the spirit world to commune with spirits on healing and other issues. In many cultures the shaman would be responsible for healing, could tell a fortune, would serve as a soul guide for the coming of a newborn or a departing soul and would keep traditions alive by memorizing songs and tales. Medicinal use of local plants is often another function of the shaman. Shamans in many cultures have additional powers over weather, crops and can use their powers to help or to hurt. Shamanism is still practiced in many cultures around the world, especially where Western medicine has limited availability or among indigenous cultures.

Shamans may inherit their abilities or title or they can be initiated by serious illness. They may be "called" to the work by being struck by lighting or similar near-death experience or they simply may have the gift to become a shaman. In today's cultures shamans often bring to mind stereotypes of witch doctors, New Age gurus or figures like Carlos Castaneda. Many areas have classes and seminars on becoming a shaman.

USER COMMENTS: *"When you're fighting cancer you'll try almost anything, which is why I found myself in Brazil sitting in front of a South*

American Indian who claimed to have healing powers. He was very well known in several countries despite the fact he didn't even have a grade school education.

"When he went into a trance he began speaking in the voice of his spirit guide, a European who'd been dead for many centuries. I was told exactly what my illness was and what needed to be done to cure it. He didn't use the same name as the medical doctors; it was more a description of what was happening in my body. I was given some crystals as a reminder of what I was supposed to do to find my healing."

(Author's note: the woman who experienced this shaman passed away less than a year later.)

"Shamanism has been around for tens of thousands of years, and thus has a huge morphogenic field around it. So it is also a powerful modality, but who is doing it is the key. Which group of healers did the practitioner study with? Does this practitioner call himself a shaman? A real shaman won't do that. A real shaman will say, 'I practice shamanism,' but never 'I am a shaman.' A good shaman can heal anything but it has to do with the healer, not the modality."

SILVA METHOD™
www.silvamethod.com

Jose Silva spent 22 years researching a wide variety of disciplines ranging from the scientific to the religious before creating his mind-training program in 1966. The **Silva Method**™ is a self-empowerment program of 16 exercises was designed to enhance the way you think and expand your awareness. It is a system, a scientific, step-by-step process of developing and using the mind effectively. It is not a religion or cult and it does not go against religion in the world, it is about helping people help themselves.

In 1989 he co-authored with Robert B. Stone *You the Healer: The World-Famous Silva Method on How To Heal Yourself and Others* about the health benefits of his method. Everything we do begins with thought, including our health. The Silva Method™ thought conditioning develops the spiritual healing which leads to mental and physical healing along with reducing stress and anxiety. Proper mental exercise is also vital for a healthy attitude and illness prevention.

The specialized 2-day Self-Healing course is one of the many Silva Method™ courses taught by Certified Silva Method™ Instructors (CSMIs) over the last 40 years. Currently Silva programs are taught in 111 countries.

USER COMMENTS: *"My husband suffered head injuries and a fractured left thigh in a terrible car accident. Before they began to operate on him the next day I prayed while putting my three fingers (a Silva technique) together. I had a hunch to call a friend of mine. Later she told me she'd used the Alpha universal mold for three consecutive nights. After only three weeks in the hospital, my husband was discharged after two successful major operations, a brain sur-*

gery and a close reduction of his left thigh fracture with the insertion of a metal plate. After this terrible event he walks with the help of only one crutch. Thank God Silva works!"

"I had a middle-aged female patient complaining of abdominal pain. The primary attending physician, thinking of acute appendicitis referred the case to me. The history, physical examination and lab work wouldn't fit the diagnosis so I went to my Silva level and scanned her. I visualized the appendix to be normal but there was a black spot in a portion of the large bowel above the appendix.

"After a few days of watching and waiting it was necessary to operate. I found that some appendices epiploicas in the ascending colon were twisted and gangrenous already. True enough, the appendix was normal. The patient had an excellent post operative course and was discharged in perfect health. To paraphrase a popular ad, 'Times like these, we need Silva.'"

SPIRITUALITY

www.csh.umn.edu

Spirituality has been wrapped up in religion for most of human history. It has significant ramifications for health whether viewed as spirituality in religion, or at the other end of the spectrum, as more of a philosophy. It is often the keystone of psychological health with a powerful, beneficial impact on the mind-body connection.

In general terms spirituality means a connection to something greater than one's self. It usually includes a sense of the meaning of life which helps us define our purpose and to make sense of the world around us. This assists the development of the values and beliefs which support our life. Spirituality also involves a sense of connection to God, Spirit or a higher power, to ourselves and others, but it also transcends this life.

Spirituality has been described as the top of the mountain, the place where all religious paths eventually meet. Some paths are easy, some are difficult, but there is no perfect or correct path. In some cases it is said to be a sense of acceptance that everything is perfect just as it is, and that life is happening as it should for the evolution of all souls.

Carolyn Myss is one of the leaders in the field of spirituality and health. Her books, CD's and appearances promote holistic methods for good health including the role of the human energy field, personal power and archetypal patterns. While "your biography becomes your biology" she says you do have the power to heal yourself.

The concept of a life force or living energy is a common belief of spirituality. While invisible to most people, many are able to see it as an aura or glowing field surrounding the body. This concept has many names, like Chi, Qi, Ki, Prana, and it runs through many healing therapies. Those who are experienced in reading auras are said to also be able to diagnose illness.

Edgar Cayce was able to see auras and it literally saved his life one day. The story goes that he was waiting for an elevator but when the doors opened he saw something was wrong. There was not a single aura around anyone in the elevator. This was very disturbing to Cayce so he waited for the next elevator. The car that he skipped suddenly crashed killing everyone on board.

The concept of spirituality and health is becoming more accepted. As one example, the University of Minnesota established the Center for Spirituality and Healing in 1995 as a prototype of integrative medicine and a model for healthcare for the 21st century.

TRAUMATIC INCIDENT REDUCTION (TIR)

www.tir.org

Traumatic Incident Reduction (TIR) was developed by California psychiatrist Dr. Frank Gerbode in 1984. It was studied as part of Dr. Charles R. Figley's "Active Ingredient" investigation of PTSD treatments at Florida State University in 1994. Based on traditional psychoanalytic theory and desensitization methods, TIR is a simple but specific procedure that helps people resolve painful events. It can even be used to work on general emotional themes, such as emotional abandonment, by using specific incidents as examples of the issue.

Whenever the mind fails to correctly process a traumatic event, it remains a raw and sensitive event in the memory which can be triggered by current experiences. The analogy has been made that it's like a scab on the mind that never heals and anything that triggers the traumatic memory knocks the scab off again. Once the sensitivity to the traumatic event is reduced then healing can take place.

The TIR process is similar to watching a movie of the traumatic incident in your mind. The professional facilitator assists the patient in viewing the event with their eyes closed. Afterwards the therapist will ask questions and the patient will respond with their eyes open. The process will be repeated over and over and each time new details or perspectives will emerge. The facilitator makes no judgments or interpretations, but rather acts as guide to control and monitor the experience. It may take from 5 to 25 viewings of the incident before the viewer starts to feel good, a process that may take from a few minutes to several hours. Normally the process lasts about 90 minutes. Severe traumas like Post Traumatic Stress Syndrome (PTSD) may take ten to fifteen sessions for relief.

The technique is normally used by psychologist and clinical social workers but it is possible to learn TIR for your own benefit. A 4-day intensive training workshop is available from the Traumatic Incident Reduction Association and an advanced degree is not required to attend.

USER COMMENTS: "*I have changed. I got back to my self and to be the person that I was before the incident. I got to see and deal with things that happened to me and sort my feelings out so I can deal with it. I learned a lot* *about myself and other people. Also I learned to not be responsible for things that others do to us, but for ones that we do to others. I also feel strongly that if I need it, help is out there, it is my responsibility to find it and live life the way I want to."*

"Yes, I have become more confident in my abilities to care for myself and my children. I realize that problems that would have left me paralyzed with fear before, I can face up to. I have learned to take things one day at a time. I know that I am a capable person and hope to never let someone else have such complete, utter control of my life again just because I am scared to be alone. It was difficult to go through all the painful memories: but somehow having done that has filled me with strength. I have great confidence in your program and especially in my therapist's application of your theories. I hope I can progress to the point where someday I can help other people, victims of domestic violence, overcome the terrible fear of having to call for themselves and their loved ones."

WHOLE HEARTED HEALING™ (WHH)

www.peakstates.com

Whole Hearted Healing™ is a therapy used by professional therapists and occasionally as a self-help technique. It is a regression process that can be done from a normal, conscious state to deal with the traumas from the past which are the source of present problems. It can also be used with EFT and other meridian therapies. In many cases EFT is actually recommended for those individuals interested in self-help. This is a powerful therapeutic technique like TIR or EMDR which can uncover very traumatic experiences which is why it should only be used under the guidance of a licensed and experienced therapist.

Typical sessions run 30-40 minutes. In general terms the process deals with the concept that we disassociate from traumatic events, they're like watching the news on TV. While this is a natural protection mechanism it leaves us with the feelings to deal with that can trigger problems in the present. Muscle testing (applied kinesiology) and energy meridians are not used in this process.

The therapist has the individual place their hand in the center of their chest to give the body the sensation of the present. Then the therapist guides the patient into their body in the past to see the event and experience it in their body, not from an outside perspective, with the focus on their hand. This type of technique can evoke powerful memories and should be done under the care of a professional therapist.

The process can be taught in minutes but a therapist requires a week of training so they're prepared to deal with all of the problems that can arise. The third edition of *The Basic Whole-Hearted Healing Manual* by Grant McFetridge and Mary Pellicer, M.D., which is the training manual for their training seminar, is available on their website.

USER COMMENTS: "*I do use WHH with good results. Clients like it because they don't have to be a big, blubbering mess to get some significant work done. I have them write a paragraph about where they are before we start and rate the level of discomfort they are in from 0 to 10. Then, at the end, the only acceptable level is a 0. I have some who are work on their own and know to bring it to 'peace, calm and light.'"*

"I had a wonderful success with a client that I have been working with for a long time, without any real significant impact—She was so stuck in a trance of unworthiness and victimhood... When I had her disengage from the mother's feelings, stay in her chest and figure out what she was feeling about her mother's feelings, we got a sensational shift. She is now making decisions for herself, standing up for herself, and making plans for opening her own business. This is a young person who was never able to support herself or make a decision for herself. It is a miracle!"

"I attended a Whole Hearted Healing training session and have had a few experiences I would like to share. The first has to do with my long time sense of hopelessness which I have felt for as long as I can remember. In one session where we were trying to connect to our white light, I had this overwhelming hopelessness leave. It has never returned. I feel like a weight has been lifted from me."

MIND CATEGORY SUMMARY

Now that you've read the Mind section you've heard the music become a little more complicated and interesting. Most of the processes in this section could've been described as falling between a simple garage rock band and a full orchestra so let's say it's something like a big jazz band. The melodies are more complex and the harmonies more rich and full.

Interestingly this is the shortest section in the book, a bridge between the physical world of the body and the world of spirit and energy. This is our consciousness, the home of our thoughts, where we interpret our lives and the world we live in. It seems appropriate because the mind seems to have one foot in the physical world and the other in the world of energy.

You've rediscovered ancient techniques like prayer and meditation and new processes like One Brain and PSYCH-K®. You can see how the Mind-Body connection functions through Mindfulness Based Stress Reduction, EMDR and many other processes. You're reminded of the benefits of humor, art and music and have learned the importance of how you think on your health and your life.

Most important you're learning about how one part of you really is connected to all the rest of you. You are a whole being of mind, body and spirit meaning that all parts must be well for true health. You can't have a troubled mind and not experience health problems eventually. Now that you've discovered so many amazing ways to help your body and your mind it's time to turn to the most fascinating part of who you are – your spirit.

Chapter 4 – Working with the Spirit or Energy

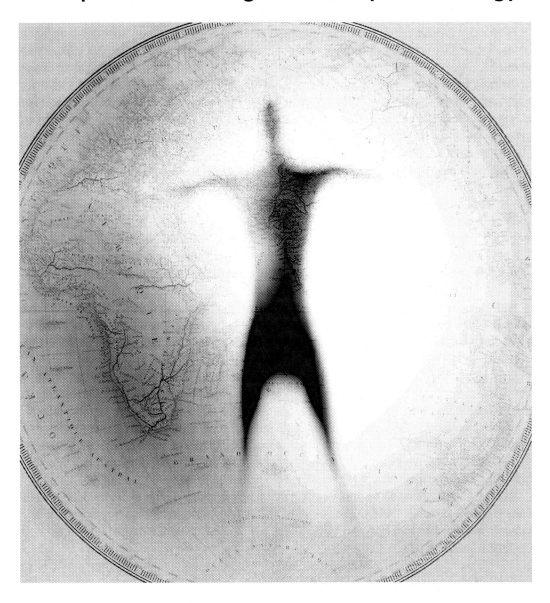

INTRODUCTION TO ENERGY/SPIRIT

Welcome to the most fascinating part of this book, the section dealing with our spirit or life energy. While it may be known by many different names in various cultures around the world throughout the history of mankind there is an almost universal belief that there is more to man and woman than simply flesh and bones. Your particular religious beliefs may provide a foundation for your perspective on this subject but you'll discover many concepts are shared through history and time. The power of prayer, for example, is recognized in religions around the world.

The subjects in this section range from the 5,000-year-old knowledge from ancient China about energy meridians to some of the most amazing scientific discoveries. You'll learn about devices that interact with the human body's biofield from Edgar Cayce's **Radiac Appliance** to a secret Russian technology developed for their space program (see **SKENAR**). You'll learn about health techniques from old-time Dowsing to the latest uses of quantum science.

As you read through this section you'll discover many common threads that run through these techniques. All of these subjects use human energy for healing, or more accurately there are many different ways to improve the flow and function of life-force energy so the body can heal itself. All believe in the indestructible nature of life energy or our spirit, and that this force can be adjusted for our benefit.

Going back to the mirror analogy again, this is where we change from a Newtonian view of the world to a Quantum-Holistic model of existence. In mainstream science the mirror is either whole or broken, one or the other. Frontier science is showing that the quantum world exists on many different levels. The mirror can be broken, whole or hundreds of variations in between and all at the same time. Our perspective of the mirror is what makes the choice as to its current state, we choose what it is.

Whether you choose to believe in prayer or cutting edge science the result is the same – a belief that the energy of life, our spirit, can change who we are and our world. In this section you'll find an amazing assortment of ideas and concepts to consider.

ACUPUNCTURE
http://nccam.nih.gov/health/acupuncture/

Acupuncture is around 5,000 years old and it is a vital part of **Traditional Chinese Medicine** (TCM). The technique stems from the belief that the body's vital energy **Chi** or **Qi** (pronounced chee) flows throughout the human body and all of nature. It consists of all essential activities meaning the spiritual, emotional, mental and physical aspects of life. Chi is composed of the universal forces of **yin** and **yang**. If the flow of Chi is low, unbalanced or interrupted, then yin and yang become unbalanced which can result in disease or illness.

Checking the **tongue** is normally the first diagnostic technique used by the acupuncturist to discover what the problems are with particular systems. In TCM, there are more than 40 different tongue types and with variations of coloring and texture, it offers a valuable diagnostic tool.

Patients will also have their **pulses** taken by the acupuncturist. Unlike Western medicine, this technique involves the differences and variations in pulses that correspond to different organs and systems. Nine spots in each wrist are examined which can take as little as five minutes or as much as thirty minutes as the acupuncturist evaluates the pulse at the top (or just under the skin), then moderately and finally by pushing down deeply.

Chi travels throughout the body along **meridians** or channels. The meridians mirror themselves in pairs on both sides of the body. There are fourteen primary meridians running vertically up and down the surface of the body. There are 12 main or organ meridians in each half of the body along with eight secondary and two unpaired midline meridians.

There are more than 2,000 acupuncture points or specific locations where the meridians come to the surface of the skin so practitioners can easily reach them with one of the nine types of acupuncture needles (but they commonly only use six in America today). The connections between acupuncture points ensure that there is an even circulation of Chi creating a balance between yin and yang. Energy constantly flows up and down these pathways but whenever the pathways become too strong, too weak, obstructed or just unbalanced, there is a problem. Acupuncture restores the balance.

Yin and yang are opposing forces that work together when balanced. Yin is usually associated with qualities that are feminine, dark, cold, moist and passive. Yang's qualities are just the opposite, being masculine, hot, dry and active. Nothing is completely yin or yang but a combination of both forces. All of this is based on the Dao or "path of life" philosophy. It is not necessary to share this belief in order for acupuncture to work!

The Food and Drug Administration (FDA) finally approved the use of acupuncture needles by licensed practitioners in 1996. These needles must be sterile, nontoxic and disposed of after a single use. They vary by length, size of the shaft and the head shape but can be as fine as a human hair. There is a wide variety of techniques used with acupuncture needles based on the patient's condition and required treatment. Doctors or practitioners can insert the needles at a low angle or perpendicular to the skin. The sensations vary by individual from almost nothing to a slight sting. Once inserted the practitioner may also manipulate the needle depending on the required treatment. The practitioner may raise or lower, rotate, scrape or in other ways manipulate the needle for the desired effect. Most people feel little or no pain when they feel the needles inserted. Reactions to treatment vary from a sensation of filled with energy to a feeling of relaxation.

Herbs are also part of TCM and often accompany acupuncture treatments. There are over 2,000 different ingredients used to customize treatment for each person's condition. Ingredients such as ginseng are mixed together to be boiled into a tea for the patient.

There are variations of acupuncture technique such as electro-acupuncture where the acupuncturist attaches clips to the needles to allow very small electrical impulses to flow into the acupuncture point. The process is safe since the amount of power used is only a few microamperes. The frequency of the current used can vary from five to 2,000 Hz based upon the desired treatment.

There are also different devices and types of acupuncture. A **Plum Blossom** is the "hitting hammer" because the device has a group of needles on its surface for a different acupuncture effect. **Acupressure** (*see listing*) is simply acupuncture without needles. The practitioner uses their hand, knuckle or a small device to stimulate the acupuncture points. There is also **Moxibustion,** which is applying heat to acupuncture points. **Cupping** is a technique that uses suction, frequently created by warming a glass cup, to draw blood to a site for stimulation.

There are also complimentary types of treatments to acupuncture. **Auricular acupuncture** involves only the points in the ear. Newer variations include using cold lasers and sound waves (**sonupuncture**) to stimulate acupuncture points.

Many researchers have conducted a variety of clinical studies on acupuncture with varying degrees of success. However, in 2005 the combined study by the National Institute of Health and The Mayo Clinic confirmed that acupuncture can help relieve the pain of fibromyalgia and can be a beneficial compliment to treatments for osteoarthritis of the knee.

There are many theories that try to explain how acupuncture works such as the Augmentation of Immunity Theory; the Endorphin Theory; the Neurotransmitter Theory; the Circulatory and the Gate Control Theories. Western medicine continues to search for a physical reason to explain how acupuncture works because Western theory does not accept the fundamental concept of a life force, the energy known as **Chi.**

China has both Western and Traditional Chinese medicine, with the masses choosing in many cases to remain with TCM while the more progressive and elite members of society choosing Western medicine. In China, practitioners use acupuncture to treat everything, even using it as an anesthesia in open-heart surgery.

America is just beginning to discover the healing potential of TCM and acupuncture. Many Americans first learned about acupuncture when James Reston of The New York Times wrote about it following his appendectomy during President Nixon's trip to China in 1971.

Acupuncture is one of the few complementary and alternative (CAM) therapies that may be covered by many insurance companies but it recommended that anyone interested in this treatment check with their carrier regarding their policy. Acupuncture treatments vary in length per session and in the number of sessions required to treat a particular condition.

According to the 2002 federal study on Americans' use of complementary and alternative therapies, more than 1% of the country used acupuncture in the 12 months prior to the survey. Four percent of those surveyed reported that they had used acupuncture at some time.

Although laws are constantly changing, currently 44 states require certification or training in order to perform acupuncture. The remaining six are Alabama; Delaware; Mississippi; North and South Dakota and Wyoming. Each of the 44 states has its own requirements and policies so it is best to research the law in your own state. For example, Oklahoma permits doctors (M.D.s and D.O.s) to perform acupuncture with no training requirement. Many recommend that you look for acupuncturists whose training has the recognition of the National Certification Commissions on Acupuncture and Oriental Medicine (NCCAOM) http://www.nccaom.org/ or the Accreditation Commission for Acupuncture and Oriental Medicine (ACAOM). See www.acaom.org

USER COMMENTS: *"Like many people, I came to acupuncture because Western medicine did not have any answers for my problems. The first time was certainly an interesting experience because I didn't know that the human tongue could have literally thousands of variations of color and texture and that each one has meaning.*

"I'd also never had a doctor take a pulse in such a strange way, lifting his fingers and moving back and forth to feel for changes and differences at different levels. It turns out they're not only evaluating the physical signs but watching for signals of the emotional health of the patient. The Chinese culture is not one to air their dirty wash in public so healers have learned to use more subtle forms of communication. Often the longer they seem to be taking the patient's pulse, they're actually learning how nervous or upset he or she is by his/her behavior.

"It's interesting how the needles feeling varies from one spot to the next and from visit to visit. One time I'll hardly feel anything at all as the practitioner placed the needles all over my body. The next visit it seems like every single one burns like crazy—like being stuck with a hot poker. Sometimes it will only be a spot or two, you just never know. There are times I have wondered if it was worth it, but the fact that acupuncture does help provides the incentive to stick to it.

"Cupping can leave an interesting collection of bruises on your back so it's best to skip the gym for a little while. Normally they'll put eight glass bowls down your back in two rows and then put candles on each one to provide the heat that creates the vacuum. I don't usually feel any of the heat, but you can usually feel the suction happening, and you can definitely feel them being peeled off. Not a painful sensation, just unusual, like so many things you experience with acupuncture.

"I've used Chinese herbs to do moxibustion, which is applying heat to acupuncture points to continue treatment. This homework was a little challenging

since the herb looked like some kind of colorful Chinese cigar and smelled like marijuana when it burned, but anything is worth it if it helps you feel better. I had to make a chart of the spots and sequence after the acupuncturist marked them on my body but after a few sessions, you learn how to do it. You should best do it outside or at least in a very big room since the aroma lasts a long time.

"Acupuncture does work! It may not be as fast as Western medicine but since it doesn't have toxic side effects I'm certainly willing to accept the trade-off of speed versus safety. After all, it wouldn't still be in use today with millions of people after thousands of years if it weren't helping. I do recommend it but have heard that some folks find the needles too painful or simply don't see any results so like with any type of medicine the patient has to realize he (or she) is responsible for his/her own health."

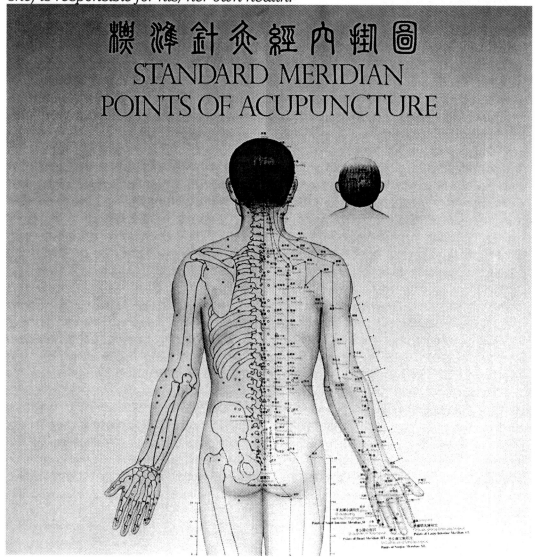

ACUPRESSURE

Acupressure, also called **contact healing**, is based on the same ancient healing principles as acupuncture and is believed the use of needles. Here practitioners use fingers, the elbow or a device to press key points on the surface of the skin to stimulate the body's natural healing abilities. Again, sickness is caused by an upset or blockage in the body's electromagnetic fields and by restoring the balance of energy you can restore health.

As with acupuncture, indicated points may not be near the diseased area, but will be on the proper point of the meridian for that particular condition. When acupressure points are pressed and it's sore then it's an indication of an energy leak at that spot. Pressing on the point closes the energy leak, releases muscle tension and promotes the circulation of blood and the body's life force energy to promote healing. As with acupuncture, more than 1 treatment may be required to reverse symptoms by allowing the body to heal itself. The biggest advantage of acupressure is that you can do it by yourself, as often as needed, simply using any one of the self-help instruction books on the market.

Auricular Therapy, also known as **ear acupuncture**, first appeared more than 2,300 years ago in China. It was widely used during the Jin Dynasty period of 265-420 A.D. to promote health and treat disease. Following the discovery by a French practitioner in 1957 that the auricular points were similar to the shape of an inverted fetus, practitioners have combined this new perspective with Traditional Chinese Medicine into **Chinese Auricular Therapy**. Continued research has added more than 200 points on the external ear which correspond to parts of the body for diagnosis and treatment. With these discoveries of new points and treatment patterns, the World Health Organization in 1982 asked the Chinese Acupuncture & Moxibustion Association to develop the International Standard of Auricular Points.

Originally, practitioners treated the ear points with needles or massage. Today there are many new ways to stimulate these points, such massage stimulation, magnets and even lasers. In some cases, practitioners may tape small beads or magnets to the ear points to provide continued stimulation for many hours and days.

Luo Points are acupressure points in the body which are believed to have special significance. These 12 points are thought to be places where the body can be manipulated to greater effect to promote the circulation of Chi to keep the body healthy.

There are different variations of traditional acupressure or ancient pressure point methods which employ varying rhythms, pressures, and techniques to create different styles of acupressure. Shiatsu is a Japanese version of acupressure and is probably the most well-known style. It can be quite vigorous, with firm pressure applied to each point for 3 to 5 seconds. **Tuina**, which is Chinese for "pushing and pulling" is similar but is more involved with soft-tissue manipulation and structural realignment. On the other hand the **Jin Shin** style gently holds each point for a minute or more.

Cupping, or fire cupping, can also be part of acupressure, and is often recommended to treat back, neck, shoulder and other muscle or skeletal pain. Variations of the process can also be found in the folk medicine practices of many countries. There have been many scientific studies which suggest the effectiveness of acupressure, particularly the wrist point known as P6 in the treatment of nausea.

There are also many other processes based on acupressure such as **Process Acupressure** which is considered a body/mind/soul modality. **Jin Shin Do**® ("The Way of the Compassionate Spirit") is a synthesis of traditional Japanese acupressure techniques, classic Chinese acupressure theory, Reichian segmental theory, Taoist philosophy and Qigong exercises. Another variation of the Jin Shin technique known as **Jin Shin Jyutsu** was brought to the West by Mary Burmeister in the 1950s.

As with other forms of Traditional Chinese Medicine (TCM) acupressure is considered to be only one part of the process. TCM always recommends that you eat a healthy diet of natural foods from soil with sufficient mineral content to facilitate the body's electromagnetic energy. Using acupressure to contact the body's nerve centers which are in trouble and using your mind constructively are also requirements for good health.

USER COMMENTS: *"The first time I used acupressure was for abdominal pain. I bought a do-it-yourself book and took it on vacation to Hawaii and it was a good thing I did! Something I ate there didn't agree with me and I woke up in the middle of the night with very painful cramping. I laid there for several minutes before grabbing my book and heading for the bathroom where I started looking up the pressure points for the problem. I tried a variety of points with varying amounts of pressure and after just a few minutes the cramping stopped when my bowels let loose of everything. I made a mental note of the points that seemed to solve the problem for future reference.*

"I've used acupressure over the years for a variety of ailments with varying amounts of success, probably related as much to my technique and the process. On many types of muscle pain it's proven very effective, as have the points for relieving nausea. I did break down and buy some of the wrist bands for a boat trip but I knew where to put them more accurately thanks to my experience.

"I've tried those so-called Shiatsu massage devices but they're like a blunt-force instrument. Acupressure is about finding the right point for the problem, not beating the entire area into submission. I guess the best analogy would be the devices tend to work like a sawed-off shotgun when the situation really calls for a small caliber handgun. Precision is the key to effectiveness.

"What I like most about it is that it can be used at any time without any equipment. It's safe, easy and can be a life-saver. I think every household should have a basic book on acupressure just like they do a first-aid guide, it's amazing how many ways it can come in handy."

"I told a practitioner friend of mine that I was tired and didn't know if I had enough energy to do what we had planned for the evening. She had her tuning forks with her so she gave me a treatment, putting the handles of the forks

against various acupuncture points on my fingers, toes wrists and ankles. She would strike them first and I could feel the vibrations. It was a pleasant sensation and when I got up I felt 'bright eyed and bushy tailed' as they say and completely ready to go! Since it usually takes me quite awhile to recover my energy after I've expended it, I found that remarkable."

ALPHABIOTICS
www.alphabioticsinternational.com

Developmental **Alphabiotics** is grounded in modern physics and the wisdom of the ages. The name derives from "alpha" meaning the first or primary principle and "biotics" which has to do with life. Fundamental Alphabiotics assumptions are: A Supreme Intelligence holds everything that exists in form and experience; each of us holds a latent spark of divinity; we are awakening Spirit beings with a mind and body; our mind is the mediator between our Source and expression; because of our misconception of reality we deal with life through an egocentric lesser self resulting in fear, stress and disharmony and the Alphabiotic Principle of Alignment/Unification is the "binding back to Source" through the Alphabiotic Process to unify the physical with the spiritual.

Alphabiotic participants explore the range of changes and positive benefits that can occur when he or she awakens from an out-reactive, egotistic state and reconnects with Spirit in a sustained way. The hands-on Alphabiotic process triggers a shift which results in changes on every level of being. The process involves a fifteen-second, hands-on procedure applied while gently cradling a person's head. As a result there is a shift to balance, strength and harmony which increase a participant's potential and ability to live life at a higher level.

Alphabiotics was introduced to the world in 1971 as a fully tested, evidence-based and scientifically grounded holistic system. The basic principles and implementing process were revealed to Dr. V. B. Chrane in the 1920s. Later his son and grandson, Drs. Virgil and Michael Chrane, continued to study, research and expand the understanding of this unique discovery. Training to become an Alphabiotics facilitator is thorough. The academic program is extensive and the skill necessary to be qualified in administering the Alphabiotic Process is comparable to training for a professional sport. No one is deemed competent until they can prove to the Alphabiotic Certification Committee that their intent is correct, that they understand and can explain basic principles and correctly administer the Alphabiotic Process.

USER COMMENTS: *"Alphabiotics has literally saved my life. If it wasn't for this science I doubt that I would be here to tell you about the changes that have happened over the past two years. If anyone feels like they just can't go on and live the life they were meant to live on earth, try Alphabiotics, it may help you more than you can imagine."*

"I feel that I am more connected to my inner Source of power, inspiration and wisdom; that I am more alive, awake and aware. Also my health is better now that it has been in twenty years."

"Through Alphabiotics, the body's own healing energy is allowed to bring about proper conditions. At the same time, since what the Alphabioticist does is so basic, the beneficial effect of any other Life enhancing activity is magnified."

AQUA CHI™ ION HYDROTHERAPY

www.aquachi.info

The **Aqua Chi Ion Hydrotherapy** device is a portable foot bath that is said to amplify the body's ability to heal as a result of a special bio-electric charge. The process is also called a detox foot bath. The device resonates in the water producing negative ions which are supposed to be similar to those found in natural hot springs. Exposure to this field through the feet is intended to re-balance the energy meridians of the body.

USER COMMENTS: *"The first time I was just amazed as the water changed, it was a very eye-opening experience and something I wanted to continue to use and explore to increase my health."*

"I've taken probably about a dozen baths and I've found that each time my energy and mental clarity improves. If I'm down emotionally or having 'one of those days' a foot bath will help clear my mind."

ASSOCIATION FOR COMPREHENSIVE ENERGY PSYCHOLOGY

www.energypsych.org

The ACEP is the professional organization for energy psychology, the collection of mind/body techniques which have demonstrated effectiveness in helping with a variety health problem. It is a nonprofit organization dedicated to unifying the many different methods of energy psychology, its promotion and the development of collaboration and cooperation among practitioners, researchers and licensing bodies.

These mind/body techniques focus on the human energy field which consists of three major, interactive systems. The first system is the series of energy pathways called meridians from Traditional Chinese Medicine. The second system is the energy centers known as chakras and the third system is the biofield, the energy that surrounds and penetrates the body.

The association also offers training for two basic types of certification in the field. The CEP.D certification or Comprehensive Energy Psychology Diplomate is for licensed mental health professionals. The EHP-C certification, Certified Energy Health Practitioner, is intended for all practitioners who successfully complete the required training and testing.

BODYTALK SYSTEM™

www.bodytalksystem.com

Dr. John Veltheim created the **BodyTalk System**™ in 1995. The Australian chiropractor and acupuncturist recognized the need to resynchronize the body's energy systems. These systems provide the communications among all of the body's systems, thus promoting the body's innate healing power. The body's life lines or communication pathways can be damaged in many ways. Problems can be caused by physical stresses, emotional traumas, chemical substances in our food and water and from exposure to artificial energy fields resulting from overhead electrical wires, cell phones, TV's, computers and other electronic equipment.

This technique is a combination of the principles of chiropractic, acupressure and kinesiology along with the ancient Hatha Yoga technique of tapping. It views the person as a whole system of mind, body and spirit. It is complimentary to traditional Western medicine and other processes or can be used as a stand-alone healing technique.

The BodyTalk practitioner uses a type of muscle testing for biofeedback to identify the problems in the body, to discover the circuits which are out of proper alignment and to find the priority of the issues. The practitioner then touches the parts that need repair while tapping the skull to focus repairs on the selected location. Tapping the skull and sternum initiates proper body communication with the problem organ or system.

Normally a BodyTalk session lasts for approximately 30 minutes, and clients usually achieve symptom relief in two or three sessions. Clients lie on a table wearing loose-fitting cotton clothing if possible. They will also remove their jewelry and belt buckles for the session.

Practitioners can cover the basic training in 38 hours of workshop time.

USER COMMENTS: *"My client was a woman in her forties. She was depressed after the death of her son, and she had developed asthma. She had to use her emergency inhaler three times a day whereas twice a week would be considered a safe dosage. She came to me because she was worried about using too much medication to control her asthma. During the first session, we found by asking Innate that she had in part inflicted the asthma upon herself. After her son's funeral, she made a garden out of all the plants and flowers she had received. This garden she had made was affecting her health because it was re-traumatizing her each time she went out to the garden. So, we treated the link between the rose garden and her lungs so that the garden would not affect her health anymore. When she came back to see me the following week, she felt much more relaxed, and she had the first positive dream about her son she had ever had since he died two years prior. In the dream, she saw her son coming through the garden and hugging her. He told her that he was doing well. This dream was a great dream. Since her final session, she has not had to use her inhaler for three months and counting."*

"An elderly man came to BodyTalk because he had been diagnosed with an enlarged left ventricle. After 7 sessions, he had a MUGA scan that showed 'the left ventricle is normal in size and demonstrates uniform wall motion at rest.'"

"A man in his 30s slipped and fell on a piece of rebar spearing his sphincter and colon. After several surgeries he developed calcified adhesions, first at the colon then further up at the duodenum. He was fed intravenously and his stomach fluids were pumped out through a tube in his neck. The hospital had sent him home, telling him that this was all they could do for him. I saw him 5 times. After 2 sessions he developed diarrhea, after the 3rd session his body literally ejected the tube from his neck and after the 5th session the doctors couldn't find the location of the blockage anymore. I never saw him again: all his functions had returned to normal."

"A 40-year-old housewife and mother who was diagnosed with MS 1-½ years ago. Her symptoms included headaches, acute hearing loss in her right ear, vertigo, and a weakness in her left leg. She was able to walk short distances but her leg weakness did not allow her to go for even a short walk. After she learned of her diagnosis, she developed panic attacks and obsessive compulsive habits (compulsive hair brushing, sock sorting and blanket folding). During a BodyTalk session linking her nervous system to her brain she suddenly opened her eyes wide and stared at me inquiring whether I was shaking her leg. She felt a strong vibrating sensation going down her left leg. Followup visits confirmed that the weakness in her leg had disappeared. Further work with the nervous system came up linking to an Active Memory that took her back to the time of the diagnosis. Her symptoms of panic and obsessive compulsive habits vanished to the point that she discontinued her anxiolytic medication."

CALLAHAN TECHNIQUES® THOUGHT FIELD THERAPY® (TFT)
www.tftrx.com

Roger J. Callahan, Ph. D. developed Thought Field Therapy (TFT) after 30 years of practice as a clinical psychologist with his wife, Joanne M. Callahan, MBA. After exhausting all standard therapy techniques with a difficult patient he realized that negative emotions were not built into the wiring of the brain or nervous system but were in a thought field of energy. This disturbance or "perturbation" could be collapsed by re-tuning the energy using the energy meridian system of the body. Originally the technique involved "tapping" selected meridians in a specific sequence or algorithm but it has evolved into a more productive process.

This process is considered the grandfather of energy psychology today. Innovations from these fundamental principles include EFT (Emotional Freedom Technique) and many variations which use different sequences or techniques. Today TFT is available as a self-help technique, by visiting trained TFT practitioners in person, or by telephone consultation. A special voice analyzer is used during the telephone interview to identify those meridians and points that need to be addressed. Nutrition is also now considered a key factor in this mental health process.

Since 1980 Dr. Callahan has written several books and appeared on many radio and TV programs about this break-through innovation in the treatment of mental and physical disorders.

Training and standards for TFT are provided by the Association for Thought Field Therapy.

USER COMMENTS: *(edited from website) "The subjects in the study were college students who identified themselves as having fear of heights. They were asked to approach and climb a four foot ladder. We hoped that the ladder was of sufficient height to provoke an acrophobic response, but not so high as to put the subject at physical risk. (After tests measuring their phobia) the experimenter treated them with either with TFT or the placebo treatment. Although both groups got somewhat better there was a statistically significant difference between those subjects who had received real TFT and those who had received placebo, with the TFT subjects showing significantly more improvement."*

"One to three Thought Field Therapy sessions were provided free of charge to individuals and families. Services were provided at the school or at home. In most cases, TFT was done in the presence of other family or community members. Algorithms were used to treat a wide range of thought fields based in memories ranging from single incidents of psychological threats to multiple acts of the worst possible violence and torture. During the first meeting clients were asked to complete a pre-test evaluating post traumatic stress symptoms. There was nearly a 40% decreased of frequency of symptoms reported overall. These results were constant across age, primary language, gender, ethnicity, and service provider."

CHAKRA ENERGY CLEANSING
www.qigongenergyhealing.com

In Hindu **Chakra** means "wheel" or "wheel of light" and it describes this vortex of energy that spins at different speeds and vibrational levels. Buddhist, Jainist and Hindu religions all consider chakras to be vital energy centers in the body. According to ancient writings there are 88,000 chakras but only the 40 secondary chakras are considered significant. Of those the seven primary chakras which are located along a vertical axis across the front of the body are vital for the body, mind and soul. Chakras for men and women spin in different, complimentary directions.

The first or lowest chakra called the root chakra is red, spinning at the slowest speed with its funnel opening to the earth. It is associated with survival and allows us to be grounded.

The second chakra is tied to emotions, creativity and sexuality. Its color is orange and it's located below the navel. The third chakra is yellow, involves personal power and self-esteem and is located in the solar plexus. The fourth chakra is known as the heart chakra. It's green, deals with love and healing, and is located near the heart over the sternum. The fifth chakra is light blue, is located at the base of the throat, and deals with communication and speaking the truth. The sixth chakra is located at the Third Eye, a spot in the center of the forehead just above the eyebrows. It can be dark blue or violet and is the focus of our imagination, clairvoyance and intuition. The highest or seventh chakra is found at the top of the head, spinning the fastest of all chakras, with a white or violet color. The Crown Chakra is about knowledge, understanding and our connection to the Divine.

These energy centers can become blocked by traumatic emotional events and stresses which impede the natural flow of energy, especially the kundalini creative energies which flow up the spinal cord. These blockages from stresses become locked into associated areas of the physical body system. Cleansing and opening chakras takes many forms. Meditation is one of the most simple but powerful methods of cleansing blockages, especially when used with visualization techniques. Colored lights, candles, oils and herbs may also be used along with mantras, chants and prayers. Various forms of energy work such as Reiki and Qi Gong may also be used to cleanse and open chakras.

USER COMMENTS: *"As with many new things, this one struck me as very weird the first time. I was using a friend's chakra clearing kit which was a small wooden box with 7 sections, one for each chakra center. There was a stone in each spot which was supposed to be sensitive to the energy of that particular chakra center. When you held a small pendulum over it the device would begin to swing in a clockwise manner which was supposed to show healthy, normal energy flow. If it circled in a counter-clockwise direction it meant that chakra was blocked and you would simply smell the essential oil that was in that section. Amazingly when you retested it just a few seconds later the pendulum would usually circle in the right way! How can a pendulum and a stone show the energy of your chakras? How does smelling an essential oil clear a blocked chakra? I don't know but it sure is fascinating!"*

"My experience was quite remarkable and I want to thank you for sharing your connection and talent with us. My experience was overwhelming physically, as well as visually. I experienced extreme heat in my thighs and especially my right thigh...then the energy moved up to the adrenal area and there was intense pain, so much that I had to do a lot of breathwork to assist the pain in moving. The whole time I felt like I was cemented to the futon and couldn't move even if I tried. My next experience was like having sandbags on my chest and this motivated more breathwork for the duration of the session. While these physical sensations were happening I was shown many visions most of them are out of reach for me at this time, however what I do remember was quite lovely."

"I continue with these sessions because they are changing me. It is not something I can enumerate such as loss weight or clearing an illness or becom-

ing stronger or any of the other types of concrete results. My results are what I call internal. Internally I am healing. I feel like I am healing from the inside out. My inside has periods of pure Joy. This is a proof of success to me. I do not think the same as I used to before these sessions, I do not react the same, I do not act the same and I am seeing both within and without differently."

CRYSTAL BOWL THERAPY or Singing Bowl Therapy
www.bestbowls.com

Crystal Bowl Therapy is a sound or vibration therapy to heal the body's energy system. Sound has been used for healing in many cultures around the world for thousands of years. Tibetans continue to use bells, bowls of crystal or brass along with other devices today as part of their religious practices. If you've ever run a wet finger around the rim of a wine glass then you're familiar with the type of vibrations a crystal bowl can produce.

This therapy is based on the concept that everything in the universe, including our bodies, vibrates at a particular frequency. Parts of your body have different frequencies so when something is vibrating out of tune or out of harmony with the rest of the body resulting from an energy blockage there is disease or illness. Using sound vibrations which are felt and heard it's possible to open the blockages and correct the resonant frequency of the chakras, meridians and other energy centers. This process is designed to restore harmony between the physical and subtle body.

Crystal bowls are made from crushed quartz that is almost 100% pure which is melted in molds. They come in a variety of sizes, often 10" to 24", to produce at least the seven tones which correspond to the seven main chakra centers. They are made to "sing" by running a device like a suede-covered mallet around the edge of the bowl.

Bowls made from brass and other materials are also used in various cultures. Their purpose is also to stimulate healing by correcting problems with the flow of life energy in the body.

These sounds are also used in mediation.

USER COMMENTS: *(with permission from www.bestbowls.com website)*
"I heard the bowls once and their effects are still with me."

"Someone brought one into our sweat lodge; it was the most powerful sweat I've ever been in."

"I felt the energy in the whole room shift and clear."

"Your bowls instantly transport me to a higher place."

"I often find my adolescent son and his friends reverently playing the bowl. What a pleasant switch from video games!"

DISTANCE HEALING

Distance Healing may encompass the widest range of concepts in the world of complementary and alternative therapies. **Prayer** may be the simplest form of distance healing but the concept is also called **Remote Healing**, **Psychic Healing, Energy Healing, Quantum Healing** and many other names. Simply put it involves the ability of mental or life force energy to impact the human body at a distance.

All of these concepts involve some type of energy manipulation. We're familiar and comfortable with energies ranging from sound to light to magnetism because there is technology which can identify and measure it. Most people are less comfortable with fields of living energy because to date there is no scientific technology which can measure bioenergy fields.

These human energies have a variety of names around the world from Qi or Chi in Traditional Chinese Medicine to Ki in the Japanese Kampo system, Doshas in Ayurvedic Medine and many others. You may know it as Prana, Etheric Energy, Vital Energy, Auras, Homeopathic Resonance or any one of a hundred different names. The fact that it's recognized in so many different cultures over thousands of years should offer credibility to the concept that human beings do have a field of living energy that penetrates and surrounds the body.

While traditional Western medicine is based on a biochemistry model, energetic medicine (also called vibrational medicine) is based on **biophysics**. In other words it's a way of correcting health problems based on quantum physics. In Europe today it's also known as regulative or virtual medicine and the concept is more accepted there than it is in America.

Diksha or **Deeksha** is another type of distance healing that is based upon the transfer of divine energy creating a neurobiological change in the brain resulting in spiritual clarity, inner calmness and a connection to the universe. In some ways it's similar to the use of prayer since it connects divine power with health. The concept is also part of Reiki.

According to reports there have been more than 150 controlled scientific studies on distance healing published over the last forty years, more than 2/3 showing positive effects.

DOWSING or Radiesthesia

www.dowsers.org

Dowsing is the use of a device to locate objects, often underground, or people. It was originally known as water witching but when used for medical diagnosis it's often called **Radiesthesia**. Dowsing is also used today for determining illness and the benefit of medicines or supplements. Pictures of forked rods appear in artwork in Egypt and China dating back thousands of years. In the Middle Ages the process was used to find coal and metals in Europe.

Devices can be a rod bent into an "L" or "Y" shape, two straight rods which cross over each other, a pendulum or other type of device. Rods are often made of brass because it conducts electricity, and therefore the electrical fields of the earth, more effectively. Some people believe the process works by reading the subtle energies of matter while others consider the technique divination or accessing our higher self. Some explain it through the **ideomotor effect** which occurs when a person unconsciously makes motions but believes it to be caused by supernatural forces, a process similar to an Ouija Board.

The technique varies by device, dowser and purpose. One style used for medical purposes is to suspend a pendulum over the patient and note the amount of swinging and direction to determine the ailment and treatment. Another method is to ask health questions and use a pendulum to receive answers. This style requires establishing which motions and directions correspond to "yes" and "no" answers initially. The amount of motion may even be rated on a scale to determine the degree of positive or negative response since some questions may have not definitive yes or no answers.

There is no licensing or certification required to become a dowser and abilities vary.

USER COMMENTS: *"The perfect and great result one can obtain when using pendulum (dowsing) to select needed homeopathic or any kind of remedy or any other kind of diagnostic and/or treatment. I used homeopathy in my practice since 1992. But only since 2005 (when I started to use dowsing in my practice) have I begun to obtain fantastic results. Moreover, I can now diagnose and treat at distance."*

"The first time I tried dowsing for health help was many years ago when my husband was still alive. My husband was having pain in his lower abdomen. I asked if it was appendicitis and got a yes. The reason I asked that question was that the pain seemed to be where my pain was when I was still in my teens. I got a yes answer and asked if we should go to the emergency room. The pain kept getting worse and I kept asking if we should go to the emergency room. I kept getting a no until about an hour later when I asked I got a yes. When we got there and finally got to see a doctor, the doctor said he must have surgery immediately. Later he told my husband that if we have come an hour earlier he would have been sent home, but that if we had come an hour later the appendix would have burst and he probably would have peritonitis and maybe died. How did it change my life? It made me trust my dowsing and I have used it every day of my life since."

"I have used dowsing to clear the aura while I am talking to someone very upset, walked around them, while still talking, then suddenly they calm down and feel great. Observers commented how great and brilliant her aura was."

EFT (Emotional Freedom Techniques)
www.emofree.com/

EFT was developed in the early 1990s by Stanford engineer Gary Craig based on the Thought Field Transfer (*TFT*) process. It's an American adaptation on the concepts of acupressure. The basic principle is that negative emotions produce an upset in the body's energy system which can be corrected by applying pressure or "**tapping**" on the major meridians. The Basic EFT process employs a comprehensive sequence of tapping points to cover all problems.

This process is unique in its openness, simplicity and eagerness to promote new forms of healing. The 87-page training manual is available as a free download from their website. While many processes are zealously guarded and tightly controlled, EFT even promotes its "cousins" on its website. There are workshops but the primary method of training is by home-study video. The basic DVD course costs $60 and there are 8 different training series available. The process is also supported by a dynamic community networked by e-mailed newsletters with testimonials and advice every few days along with media promotion to help develop consumer awareness and acceptance.

Because it is based upon the energy system in Traditional Chinese Medicine the process has been quickly accepted and its popularity is exploding. The endorsements of a variety of medical professionals have also increased its acceptance. From serious issues like Post-Traumatic Stress Syndrome to helping golfers improve their scores, their motto is "try it on everything".

Tapping, as it's also called, uses the fingertips to tap on 14 different points on the body to stimulate all of the major energy meridians. The Basic Recipe is called a ham sandwich of steps: Set-Up; Basic Sequence (13 steps); 9 Gamut and then another round of Basic Sequence. The entire process usually takes less than 2 minutes and can be learned very quickly. Follow-up rounds of EFT may be abbreviated with various shortcut routines using modified Set-Up and Reminder phrases. This process is designed for people to use by themselves but there are many experienced facilitators available for more challenging problems, either in person or by telephone.

In 2006 EFT claimed to have more than 100,000 practitioners and features an Advisory Board with several physicians. Their website is also careful to note: "While EFT has produced remarkable clinical results, it must still be considered to be in the experimental stage and thus practitioners and the public must take complete responsibility for their use of it. Further, Gary Craig is not a licensed health professional and offers EFT as an ordained minister and as a personal performance coach. Those who want to discuss the use of EFT for a specific emotional problem with a professional in the mental health field are referred to our Referral section, where a number of licensed practitioners who use EFT in their practices are listed."

USER COMMENTS: *"What's surprising is the simplicity of EFT. It really only takes a few times through to memorize the contact points in the Basic Rec-*

ipe. The basic concept of sending energy down the body's meridians in order to reboot the system seems like a practical way to solve the problem of negative energy which can come from feelings, thoughts or memories. As fascinating as it is to watch the DVDs and see how EFT affects someone else, it's even more amazing to use it yourself. It really can be used on almost anything! From emotional issues to physical problems, EFT has some amazing healing properties."

(From website) "I have tried your technique, with a lot of skepticism at first, as it defies all logic. It worked....not only the first time on my headache, but the second time on my stiff neck and tension headache, the third time on my inability to sleep, and so on."

"I tried it on myself and shot a game of golf 12 strokes under my previous best game ever."

"I have used EFT on myself and family members for a variety of quick therapies from shoulder pain to headaches, nausea, and so on. This method is absolutely invaluable."

"I have applied EFT 70 or 80 times and I have yet to come across a client who is not happy with the results EFT has given."

"We are very excited about this EFT program. My wife got rid of her back pain and too frequent headaches she has had for years. I no longer have acid reflux and no longer have to take a prescription drug for it."

EFT VARIATIONS or Other Energy Meridian Techniques

The **Active Choice Technique** (ACT) was originally called the ACUPRESSURE CHAKRA TECHNIQUE and was one of six variations on EFT developed by Dr. Philip Friedman. This style blends energy, spiritual and personal development techniques to reduce psychological and/or emotional distress. The first step is for the client to clearly focus on the emotional distress/trauma and then put one hand over their heart and the other on one of 6 selected areas of their body which are located near a chakra. The client then proceeds with the other steps in the process while repeating a series of statements designed to heal the origins of the problem along with associated issues of forgiveness or other grievances.

Creating And Receiving Technique (CART) is designed as a process for empowerment to resolve personal problems. The initial step is for the person to breathe gently while placing his or her hands near the two chakra energy centers of the chest/heart area and solar plexus. A series of affirmations are spoken with the eyes closed to release the past and affirm the present. The person then makes choices in 10 core areas of their life such as health and forgiveness while visualizing their goals in these areas.

Healing and Release Technique (HEART) is another EFT variation to help clients connect to their heart after discovering emotional barriers or limiting beliefs. While touching their heart and solar plexus to connect to chakra energy the client uses visualizations to release emotional distress. The client then visualizes light flowing into their head and circulating through the heart to promote peace and healing.

Light Imagery Grateful Heart Technique (LIGHT) is a process to focus on positive resources to promote healing and growth. It is a variation of the HEART technique where the facilitator has the client experience all of the blessings in their life. This technique is recommended for regular client use because what you focus on expands.

Miracle Acupressure Tapping Technique (MATT) has the client rubbing certain spots to stimulate the energy meridians in the body while repeating affirmations followed by focusing on the problem and finally while engaged in a forgiveness procedure.

Tap and Soft Touch Energy Technique (TASTE) is another EFT variation by Dr. Friedman that has the client rubbing a spot on the upper chest and then tapping on other meridians while thinking about the problem followed by healing affirmations. In this technique the client may hum a tune or move their eyes while tapping and working through a forgiveness process. Dr. Friedman is also the Executive Director of the Foundation for Well-Being and the author of several books and articles on energy healing. http://www.integrativehelp.com/

AER, or **The Next Step**, was created by Robert Vibert following five years of research and development. The term stands for **A**wareness, **E**xpression and **R**esolution which are the key features of the process. Built on a foundation of EFT it uses elements of deep focus, goal-building along with features from yoga and other energy techniques. The process is used by trained healers.

Many therapies are incomplete, leaving parts of the emotional wounds so this process was created to deal more thoroughly with each necessary step in the process of healing. Awareness of the real problem, not just symptoms, is the first step followed by an effective expression of the problem and finally a proper resolution. http://www.vibert.ca/nextstep.html

USER COMMENTS: *"Your approach to our process was confident, competent and compassionate. It was gentle while clearly directed. I refer to "our process" because, though you were leading, I felt throughout this healing that we were partners. You calmly yet firmly guided me through each step."*

"Robert started by asking me a question that leads me to the feelings underneath all the anger that was on the surface. After using the AER technique for 10 minutes or so, the problem with my wife dissolved, along with a long time wound from when I was six years old."

BeSetFreeFast or BSFF is an acronym for Behavioral and Emotional Symptom Elimination Training For Resolving Excess Emotion: Fear, Anger, Sadness and Trauma. It is an energy therapy developed by Larry P. Nims, Ph.D. to deal with the deep emotional sources of emotional problems. The process involves no physical contact (no tapping) and works by the power of intention using a single algorithm. His original process involved a 4-step tapping algorithm but evolved to be a non-contact technique of intention. It is designed as a self-help process to be learned by book, DVD or workshop. As with similar energy therapies the services of trained professionals are also available to assist with issues. http://www.besetfreefast.com/

USER COMMENTS: *"As a therapist and trainer of over 26 years' experience, I can honestly say that using BSFF has changed my life, and changed my therapy practice in ways that I could never have dreamed of. Over the last several years I've learned as many of the new therapies as I could, and there is NOTHING that works as fast as BSFF."*

"Wow...I cannot believe the shifts I've gotten in my own life in just a few days by applying what I learned in your book and DVDs! I've been released from layer upon layer of stuff about my parents dying young and so should I, heart attack worries, stressing about being late, the need to confront, controlling my wife, etc., etc.. This is the most amazing psychotherapeutic methodology I've ever seen (and feel free to quote me anytime). It really is simpler, more effective and goes deeper than anything I've ever been exposed to, despite years as a therapist and over 30 years in full-time hypnosis."

Conscious Healing and Repatterning Therapy (CHART) was developed by Paula Shaw, CADC, by combining traditional therapy concepts with features of the most effective energy psychology techniques. The process is based on the concept that unresolved childhood trauma interrupts normal development. People have blocked energy systems because they can't clear them only as adults, they need to listen to their Inner Child and deal with the source of the problem. The technique uses Intention, Muscle Testing, Keywords, Visualization along with Chakra and Meridian contact to clear emotional issues held by the Inner Child, the Inner Adolescent and the Adult Self. It works by correcting the Biofield, Chakras and the body's energy Meridians. http://www.paulashaw.net/

Getting Thru Techniques are a group of processes that combines features of EFT, Holistic Hypnotherapy, NLP and other processes developed by Phillip and Jane Mountrose. GTT not only helps you become aware of your physical, emotional and spiritual conditions but allows you to go deeper into your unconscious mind. The techniques are designed to release fears, unresolved emotions and other limitations as you come into contact with your subpersonality who is experiencing the difficulties.

Books, videos and classes are available for the process. Certification is done by the Awakenings Institute in California, a non-profit religious organization. http://www.gettingthru.org/egtt.htm

Healing Energy Light Process created by Dr. Fred P. Gallo combines different techniques including Educational Kinesiology, Brain Gym, yoga breathing, HeartMath and Dr. Gallo's **NAEM** process. The process focuses the patient's intention to achieve the desired outcome. It is designed to treat problems in a holistic manner which offers benefits but more focused treatments like NAEM/MET or EDxTM™ may be used as a follow-up. It can be used as part of a therapy session or clients may use it for self-treatment.

EDxTM™ is another process addressing the relationship between our emotions, conscious thoughts, behaviors and our health because all of these interrelated systems involve energy or biofields. It diagnoses the energetic problem by muscle testing and prescribes treatment. It has special techniques for dealing with psychological reversals and neural disorganization. EDxTM is not limited to meridian-based treatments. The method also includes processes such as Orientation to Origins (OTO) ™; Basal Energy Analysis and Management (BEAM) ™; diagnosing and treating introjects; and using processes, such as music and poetry, to access psychological health.

ECT™ is composed of 12 different techniques which integrate principles of consciousness, thought recognition and energy psychology. It involves working with higher consciousness so the interaction between therapist and customer becomes the catalyst for change. The process uses principles of energy and mind-thought-consciousness related to the individual's issues. See www.energypsych.com

USER COMMENTS: *"Energy Consciousness Therapy (ECT)™ is a communication and therapeutic methodology that integrates principles of consciousness, thought recognition, and energy psychology. It is based on the assumptions that mental health is innate, that energy and consciousness are integrally interrelated, that the health of the therapist is imperative to achieving positive therapeutic results, and that elevating thought recognition supports mental health and therapeutic results.*

"Aside from employing a number of energy psychology techniques, ECT™ emphasizes accessing innate health and higher consciousness so that the interaction between therapist and client becomes the primary impetus for change work. The therapeutic process conveys principles of energy, mind, thought, and consciousness that are relevant to the individual's specific issues. Through this deeper level of understanding, the problem can be transmuted and higher levels of consciousness and mental health can be maintained. Elevating the individual's level of consciousness in this way also serves to balance bioenergy."

Positive Energy Therapy (PET), **Mindful Meridian Therapy** (MMT), and **Whole Life Healing**™ (WLH) are EFT variations developed by Stephanie Rothman, Cht. Her basic concept is that if what we focus on expands, then we should focus on what's right, what's good, what's healing and what's healthy. All of her techniques also carry the philosophy of personal responsibility. http://www.lets-talk.com/?section=14

Whole Life Healing removes blocks and limitations from an individual's entire life. The preferred method is with the energy of two people in the practitioner's office.

USER COMMENTS: *"You can't imagine my reluctance about trying your Whole Life Healing technique on my fear of heights. But it worked—quickly and easily! I felt sighs of relief during the process and a sense of peace after. I've confirmed the results with a zero-blind field-test at the shopping mall—a multi-tiered open pit with disorienting glass/chrome/mirrors, glass elevator, crowds bumping victims ever-closer to a precipice—an acrophobe's spookus maximus.*

To my amazement, I could even do a skywalk from one balcony to another without cringing and tottering in the middle of the pathway. Thank you, thank you!"

"We used Whole Life Healing over two months ago to help with her food compulsions. She loved the session and has had a dramatic change in her relationship with food ever since. She simply no longer uses it to fill herself up emotionally or to stuff her feelings. She has really had to adjust to this and the changes are rippling through her life."

Mindful Meridian Therapy is an easy technique for removing perceived negatives.

Positive Energy Therapy is another easy to use and teach healing technique. This variation is for expanding healthy beliefs, habits or circumstances to attract desired outcomes.

Quantum Techniques by Stephen Daniel, Ph.D. and Beth Daniel, M.A., Ed.S have combined elements of various mind-body-spirit techniques with their own innovations into this system (*see separate listing*).

Relationship Energy Repatterning (RER) uses EFT, kinesiology, NLP and hypnosis to change life force energy that can be producing unhealthy patterns of behavior into healthy patterns of attitude, choice and behavior. The technique involves five procedures for clearing patterns and was developed by Layne and Paul Cutright. http://www.paulandlayne.com/howwework.htm

REMAP was developed by Dallas psychotherapist Steve Reed in 1997. The process is built on a foundation of EFT but capitalizes on all of the acupuncture/acupressure meridians and treatment points along with brain balancing eye movement techniques and other protocols to relieve emotional distress and limiting beliefs in the mind-body system. The synergetic effect also promotes emotional freedom further growth along life's path. See http://www.psychotherapy-center.com/the_remap_process_toc.html

USER COMMENTS: *"I personally experienced the profound and far reaching effects of the REMAP process at the training session in Richardson, Texas as Steven Reed demonstrated the technique on me. In a short period of time he brought me through an old childhood trauma. In that short period of time he was able to help me locate it, experience it and heal it very quickly. The effects have held and the emotions connected to it have been cleared. I have never experienced anything working this deeply and this fast."*

"Ever since the day after we all took the REMAP Course, I've been using it with my patients, with great results!! Every single patient that has agreed to try REMAP has improved. That's quite an achievement. I wanted to share this with you, and thank you for sharing your knowledge with us."

Seemorg Matrix Work™ is a new integrative, transpersonal therapy developed by Nahoma Asha Clinton, MSW, PhD. Using the movement of energy through the chakras, it provides lasting, thorough treatment for PTSD, negative beliefs, OCD and other anxiety, personality and dissociative disorders. It also treats allergies and physical illness caused by emotional issues. In treating spiritual blockages and developing positive attributes it opens and expands spiritual development. Clinicians also use this therapy to transform negative character structures into positive ones. www.SeemorgMatrix.org

USER COMMENTS: *"I've both received and provided Seemorg Matrix work. For myself, I've felt very powerful emotions as I'm doing the work, often memories just come by so fast in my mind that I can't stop them. Of course, they have to do with the healing that is taking place. And the SUDs level (Subjective Unit of Distress) comes down so fast with this work!*

"For my clients, when I muscle test (energy test) them, 99.9% of the time, when I ask the question: Which modality will be the quickest, easiest and provide the deepest healing it comes up Seemorg. There are just amazing results for my clients with this work."

Thought Energy Synchronization Therapy® or **TEST** is a combination of energy meridian therapy, applied kinesiology and other techniques to help therapists deal more effectively with clients.

The therapist has the client tune into the disturbing thought or memory and begins the session by muscle testing for proper biomagnetic alignment. It's not uncommon to discover polarity reversal when dealing with negative thinking. Once the client is prepared a diagnostic procedure determines the specific sequence of meridians to be stimulated for the treatment. The process was developed by Gregory J. Nocosia, Ph.D., B.C.F.E., a licensed psychologist and originator of TEST® Dx and ThoughtWorks®. www.ThoughtEnergy.com

The **Transformational Healing Method**™ (THM) was developed by Marilyn Gordon, BCH, CI as a synthesis of hypnotherapy and EFT. It increases the therapist's ability to use the subconscious mind, higher consciousness and the patient's energy system for greater physical, emotional and spiritual healing. As a comprehensive process it has the power to transform darkness in the patient's life into light. www.hypnotherapycenter.com

USER COMMENTS: *"The Transformational Healing Method™ (THM) is fabulous. I have had clients tell me that I 'saved their life,' and it was because of this method. It allows you to more easily work with almost any client, without having to start out with scripts, and the clients can receive tremendous transformational healing. The method supports, and goes beyond, regression and suggestions. My clients are having wonderful, outstanding, life-changing transformations!"*

"Even though I love hypnosis, I always felt there was a piece missing. Since your THM course, I have worked with 5 clients this past week. The experiences were amazing. Each client is so different, as you know, and their experience through transformation was beautiful to watch and share. The clients are so enthusiastic, and can't wait for their next sessions. Without exception they are thrilled, have expressed to me that they feel they have 'awakened' to life in a new way. So, thank you, thank you, thank you. I now know I have found the missing pieces I sensed I needed."

WHEE stands for Wholistic Hybrid of EMDR and EFT. It was developed by Daniel J. Benor, M.D. to work more quickly than the more proven EMDR technique. He began using the technique with children because managed care allowed a few precious minutes extra and he's expanded the success for use with parents at the same sessions. Today it can also be a self-help technique. He's continued to evolve the process by using abbreviated acupressure points found in Matrix Therapy. See www.WholisticHealingResearch.com

USER COMMENTS: *"WHEE has been working very well for my fear of riding in a car. I'll admit I was skeptical that something that sounded so easy would actually work at all, never mind so well. I really want to thank you for giving me this tool to use. You've shown me a way to access my own inner strength and inner being easily and effortlessly to deal with my phobia, and even my every-day kind of stresses."*

"Since adolescence I had suffered from performance and public speaking anxiety. Every therapy failed to relieve the burden. It was an incident in 7ᵗʰ grade that Dr. Benor and I worked on during the workshop. Although I still struggle in part from these anxieties, my experience with Dr. Benor and WHEE, and continuing practice has dramatically lessened their impact on my life."

EMOTRANCE

emotrance.com

Emotrance is a technique to heal the human energy system. Disturbed emotions like stress, anger, grief, or anxiety all come from a disturbed energy system which leads to disturbed thinking and eventually to physical disease. When you feel positive, motivated and full of joy then you feel that your energy system is working correctly.

In this process energy healing and spiritual healing may be considered the same basic concept because Emotrance is said to be a simple process built on the principles of Sacred Geometry. It deals with the movement of energy in, through and out of the body and provides a practical and theoretical framework for all types of energy healing. This process is an evolution of the basic EFT concept offering additional benefits and overcoming the inherent limitations of EFT. With Emotrance the conscious mind does not have to be aware of the specific problem. The process is able to work in wider areas because it isn't dealing only with specific energy meridians but with the entire energy body. Another major difference is that it does not involve any "tapping" or touching since it uses only the hands of the energy body for healing.

The process was developed through 25 years of research in the United Kingdom by Dr. Silvia Hartmann with assistance from Nicola Quinn. It was unveiled at the Oxford Energy Therapies Conference in Great Britain in 2002.

USER COMMENTS: *"EmoTrance is the only one which has made significant shifts in my spiritual, emotional, mental, and physical condition: from heaviness to lightness; from depression to joy, from fatigue to high energy. It is an amazing experience of just how good you can feel, how much more powerful you can be and how much more there is waiting—just for you. I want to sing and dance* *and shout to the world, 'Hey everybody, hear this. Come and truly enjoy life. Come alive. Look, what a magical world we are living in. We are in paradise.'"*

"A new client of mine had already spent about £2000 over six months at an expensive clinic with a whole range of nutritional supplements and hadn't improved at all. In fact, she said she felt worse. She'd suffered illnesses most of her life but since moving her fatigue and fybromyalgia symptoms had worsened. I asked her how she felt about being here. She said "I don't feel welcome, don't feel a part of any groups or community here". I asked her when did she first start getting ill, she said... "I've been ill all my life". Emotional charge intensified as she revealed that her Mother never wanted her, so she'd always felt unwelcome. I asked her where she felt this in her body. She said in her heart. We used EmoTrance to focus in, softening this energy and it released through her body and left through the arms and the legs. Energy also flowed up through the head, seemed to get stuck there so we softened it some more to release it all. As all this energy was releasing, the client said she was experiencing joy for the first time in so many years and that she felt 'wonderful' and couldn't remember the last time she felt this good with so much more energy. This was one session. She was by no means healed completely. A few weeks later she said that the session had made a quantum leap forward in her general well being, cheerfulness, being able to get up brighter in the mornings and feel refreshed now after sleeping. Although she still has more work to do she can now see how her emotions, and the blocked energy underlying it, can affect her physical health."

AIM Program of Energetic Balancing

www.energeticmatrix.com

AIM Program of Energetic Balancing believes that imbalances in energy impede the flow of the life force of energy. Their All Inclusive Method (AIM) Program of Energetic Balancing provides balancing energies to help you remove your own imbalances. They do not claim to heal you, rather it is a tool for clients to use for healing themselves.

This is a spiritual process performed by exposing a participant's photo to subtle-energy balancing frequencies. The photograph is considered to be part of your spiritual hologram so when your photograph is exposed to these balancing frequencies, you receive these energies. You can then use the energy to help manifest your intention to heal yourself and raise your consciousness.

Stephen Lewis, Evan Slawson and Roberta Hladek formed EMC[2] in 1998 as a spiritual technology to assist in removing energy imbalances. Mr. Lewis has degrees in acupuncture and homeopathy and is co-author of *Sanctuary: The Path to Consciousness*. Mr. Slawson has studied hatha, kundalini and ashtanga yoga along with shamanism, Reiki and hypnotherapy and is co-author of *Sanctuary*. Ms. Hladek is a student of Oriental healing arts. She also has a degree in homeopathy.

ENERGY HEALING or ENERGY WORK

Energy healing or **energy work** are generic terms describing the use and/or manipulation of life force energy (qi, chi, prana, spirit, etc.) to improve health. Types of energy healing include Reiki, chakra balancing, aura cleansing, energy field clearing, Healing Touch, Polarity Therapy, Pranic Healing, Quantum Touch, Therapeutic Touch and many other processes. For more information please see individual listings.

As noted in other chapters there are a variety of means to manipulate the living energy of human beings. These may include devices for controlling light, sound, magnetism along with the use of hands in order for the life force of the practitioner to modify the energy of the client. Hands may be used in contact or above the body. The goal of all techniques is to remove blockages and improve the flow of life energy which will lead to improved health and personal growth.

ENERGY PSYCHOLOGY

www.energypsych.org, theamt.com

Many of the therapies viewed as **energy psychology** are based on the premise that everything in the universe is composed of energy, including human beings. Some concepts consider these energy fields to be similar to the electromagnetic fields around an electrical wire, meaning the energy in our nervous system radiates a living energy field or biofield in, around and through our bodies. Throughout the history of man techniques have been developed all over the world that use this life force energy for healing. The use of this energy for psychology merges Eastern understanding of who we are with Western concepts of psychotherapy. Roger Callahan is generally credited with developing the first form of energy psychology (*see listing for the Callahan Method or TFT*) in the 1980s in California.

Explanations for how these therapies work varies from modifying the brain's electrochemistry to differences in how and where our memories are stored. Some concepts hold that memories and knowledge are stored in cells all over the body as a matter of efficiency and safety and that changing how the energy communicates this information through the body's meridians corrects problems. Other concepts are more holistic, explaining that our energy frequencies are the source of problems so correcting the frequencies or energy blockages enables healing.

There are as many different explanations as there are techniques. While many energy therapies make no claim of scientific verification, there are often parallels with the principles of quantum physics and developing fields like string theory.

The term **Energy Psychology**® is registered by Gallo & Associates Psychological Services in Europe but the term has been used to describe a variety of energy healing processes. Individual Gallo therapies include EdxTM™, NAEM™ and ECT™. (*See* **EFT Variations** *for more information.*)

FENG SHUI or Geomancy

www.InternationalFengShuiGuild.org

The term **Feng Shui** comes from "wind" (feng) and "water" (shui). More than 2,000 years ago in China it was believed the life force energy (chi) is dispersed when it rides the wind and stops when it meets water. The ancients wanted to collect and retain chi to improve their luck, success, health and their lives. The technique is the placement and arrangement of space to achieve harmony with the environment. It is not a decorating style but a discipline compatible with many types of decorating styles.

The foundation concepts of Feng Shui are: the landscape of locations; the shape of buildings; capturing chi; deflecting negative energy; applying the concept of the five elements (wood, fire, earth, metal and water); balancing yin and yang; understanding symbolism; using compass directions to define space and updating time changes. There are several different schools of Feng Shui including: the **Land Form School**; **Flying Star**; **Eight Mansions**; **Black Hat Sect**; **Nine Star Ki**; **Four Pillars** and the **Compass School**.

To have good Feng Shui means a location in harmony with nature while bad Feng Shui is to be out of place or fit poorly with nature. Feng Shui prefers rounded edges over sharp angles, for example. People are usually not described as have good or bad Feng Shui but their force of personality or even their appearance may be able to add or subtract from the Feng Shui of their surroundings.

The International Feng Shui Guild originated in 1999 as a community to promote the ancient art and science of Feng Shui. Training and certification is available as is membership for practitioners agreeing to support the association's code of conduct and standards.

USER COMMENTS: *"I had some very unruly neighbors. Their trash blew in my yard, the kids were left to themselves and they frequently destroyed small trees in the neighborhood. Their loud parties were a pretty much constant on the weekends. My Feng Shui advisor suggested I place small mirrors, round, two inches in diameter in all the windows that faced this neighbor. It took about three weeks, but they decided all on their own to build a tall fence to separate their home from mine. It was competed five weeks later."*

"My home office is now open, functional & beautiful! My business has increased and I am now proud to have clients here. Generally, I am much more relaxed & productive when before I was cramped, unorganized &stressed."

"After working in the mortgage business for 2-½ years, I was closing approximately 5 loans per month. The first month after my Feng Shui office consultation, I closed 10 loans. The next month I closed 15 loans making me # 1 in sales 2 months in a row!"

GEM THERAPY also Crystal Therapy
www.gemisphere.com

Gem Therapy has its roots in ancient cultures as diverse as Ayurveda, Chinese medicine, and Native American shamanism. It is another type of holistic therapy which focuses on the person as a whole instead of being preoccupied just with symptoms. The goal of this therapy is to restore balance and wholeness of mind, spirit and body.

The basic tenets are that human beings are unique, interconnected fields of energy and that blockages of our energy flow result in illness and disease. Each type of gemstone expresses a different frequency of energy which can be used to address different types of blockages to restore energy flow and health.

For example, according to ancient texts Ruby can improve emotional stability such as healing from painful and suppressed emotions and is good for the heart, spleen and hypertension. Green gems like Emerald are beneficial for supporting the immune system and Blue Sapphire can clear the mind, restore mental balance and help strengthen weak bones and nerves and increase vitality. Gemstone energy can be used on specific energy centers like the chakras or acupressure points or to treat the whole energy system.

Gemstones are thought to be intense concentrations of energy because they were formed over eons, often under extreme pressure. The shape of a gemstone affects its ability to express energy. The ideal shape is a sphere because it can radiate its power evenly in all directions. To be effective stones must also have no impurities to contaminate the energy and they must be of therapeutic quality. While there are over 100 gem therapy protocols reported it is possible to obtain benefits simply by wearing therapeutic gems around the neck.

Another innovation and variation of gem therapy is **Electronic Gem Therapy** which uses gemstones in lighting devices. By using colored light energy it's possible to deliver specific energy to selected parts of the body. Lamp therapy is even being used by veterinarians in some parts of the world.

Crystal Healing is a variation of gem therapy that uses natural crystals. Different colored crystals radiate different frequencies of energy which can be used for healing, for strengthening the body and resolving issues. (See also *Crystal Bowl Therapy*.)

USER COMMENTS: *"In my healthcare practice, I have found that many of the people I treat have a tremendous and heartfelt resonance with therapeutic gemstones. The effects of the gemstones are powerful. Clinical treatment with gemstones often results in profound and lasting improvements in my clients' physical and inner health, changes that clearly manifest in their everyday lives. My experience has borne out the value of these tools over and over again."*

HEALING FROM THE BODY LEVEL UP (HBLU)
www.jaswack.com

Healing From The Body Level Up is a holistic therapy system to heal a person at the conscious, unconscious, body and soul levels simultaneously. It is designed to clear mental, emotional, physical or spiritual blocks in the flow of life energy.

The mind/body/spirit healing system was developed by Dr. Judith A. Swack, a Ph.D. biochemist and immunologist. It is a synthesis of many processes including NLP, energy psychology, Applied Kinesiology, psychology and spiritual practices. It is based on the belief that we have a radiant and beautiful soul placed in this life to make a contribution to the world and that we are destined to experience the fullness and joy of life. Failure to achieve these goals results from interference from life experience, personality structure or external interference.

The process is based upon muscle testing which allows the client's deepest wisdom to dictate the goals and healing steps necessary. Information about the particular type of interference, where it's located in the body and which balances or interventions are best to clear it are included. The process also includes techniques for clients to use between sessions to resolve difficulties on their own. Some of its unique features are: the process heals on all four levels at the same time; it has a menu of standardized damage patterns to work from; it employs quick and effective techniques and as a result of its use of muscle testing it is unique to the individual.

USER COMMENTS: "*Before (my sessions) I wasn't just afraid of flying. I was petrified and unable to fly and skeptical that anyone could help, because nothing else had worked for me. Now, after just 3 sessions with you, my phobia is completely gone. I flew to New York, and although it was a turbulent flight, I was more comfortable than my flying companion.*

"*I had just heard that my company had lost a major contract and I was experiencing a loss of confidence in my team of people as well as a general "freezing up" of my creative problem-solving abilities. In just 10 minutes, Dr. Swack's techniques enabled me to unfreeze and open my mind to insights, restoring my confidence and ability to seek solutions.*

"*Next month will be the one year anniversary of my ability to resume a normal life thanks to your miraculous treatment for unlocking my physical disability resulting from a serious car accident. After a year of being unable to work, I was only able to return part time because of the physical limitations and the amount of time I spent pursuing treatment. After 45 minutes of working with you, all the pain released. My life is happier, brighter and a much more enjoyable place to be.*"

HEALING TOUCH

www.HealingTouchInternational.org

Healing Touch is a nurturing energy therapy based on the belief that everyone has the capacity to heal through touch and compassionate intent. The technique can be used for all ages and conditions of health or illness, even for animals.

By assisting in the balance of your physical, emotional and spiritual well-being, Healing Touch works with the body's energy field to support your natural ability to heal. The process uses light touch to balance and strengthen the energy field. Research has shown the process effective in improving relaxation, improving the patient's sense of well-being, decreasing pain, reducing side-effects of cancer treatments and providing a feeling of a positive change in energy.

The process was developed by Janet Mentgen, RN in Colorado during the 1980s. She founded Healing Touch in 1989 as a program of continuing education for nursing professionals and lay people interesting in healing. Today it is used in hospitals, hospices, spas and a variety of settings. She was honored in 1988 as the holistic nurse of the year by the American Holistic Nurses' Association (AHNA) for her work.

Healing Touch became a certificate program of the AHNA in 1990 and was then transferred to Healing Touch International, Inc. which was created in 1995 to certify Healing Touch Practitioners and Instructors and to promote Healing Touch worldwide. The Healing Touch Certificate Program progresses from beginner to advanced practitioner level using a variety of hands-on techniques through five levels of education.

USER COMMENTS: *"My pain level dropped from unbearable to manageable in just one session.*

"After a Healing Touch session, I feel more focused and motivated, and have a lot more energy. The cancer diagnosis was terrifying. After Healing Touch I was calm and able to function again.

"During the session, I feel tingling and warmth. Afterwards I am rejuvenated and have a sense of purpose and spiritual connection."

JIN SHIN JYUTSU®

jsjinc.net

The Art of Jin Shin Jyutsu® harmonizes the body's life energy. In Japanese the term means "art of the Creator through compassionate man". It is an ancient form of healing which was passed down by word of mouth that nearly became extinct until it was revived by Master Jiro Murai in the early 1900s. His student Mary Burmeister brought the knowledge to the U.S. in the 1950s.

The process is based on the concept of 26 energy locks along energy pathways in our bodies. As with Chinese acupuncture, whenever these paths become blocked the energy flow is disrupted resulting in disharmony, illness and disease. It can be applied as a self-help process or by a trained practitioner. It does not involve massage or manipulation.

Sessions usually last about one hour with the person lying fully clothed face up on a soft surface or massage table. The session begins with the taking of pulses, or listening to the energy flow in the wrists. The practitioner will then use a harmonizing sequence of hand placements called a "flow" to unblock particular pathways by using gentle fingertip or hand contact to stimulate energy circulation. Because each person and session is unique there is no systematic technique, each process is customized, which is why it is called an art. The process also reduces tension and stress by releasing blocked energy and restoring normal flow.

Training and certification is done by Jin Shin Jyutsu, Inc. in Scottsdale, Arizona.

USER COMMENTS: *"My friend had a twenty-year history of asthma. I showed her how to hold her ring fingers to strengthen her respiratory functions. She remarked on being able to breathe more freely after holding them and decided to receive some Jin Shin Jyutsu sessions from me. I focused on balancing the second depth. After three sessions, she said she felt like a new person. She didn't need any medication or vaporizers since receiving Jin Shin Jyutsu. Also, she said she could feel her lungs become more clear for the first time.*

"Recently I was on a business trip and I stepped off of a curb and landed one foot in a pothole. It really hurt when it happened but I just walked it out (or so I thought). Many hours later, after a long flight home and walking miles from the airport terminal to my car, I got home and removed my shoe. The moment I removed that shoe, my foot began to swell and hurt so bad that I could not even walk on it. I was in such pain that I immediately called my friend for some Jin Shin Jyutsu. She started by putting her right hand down and the left hand on top of it for the swelling, and I felt the heat rushing out of my foot. Then she did a Bladder flow and a #15 release flow which had me sleeping within twenty minutes. I am always amazed at the power of Jin Shin Jyutsu...from incredible pain to sound asleep in twenty minutes! I have never gotten that kind of result from anything else. Because of Jin Shin Jyutsu, I was able to walk to a very important meeting the next day, all of the soreness was gone. Remarkable!"

KOREAN CHI THERAPY

http://www.lime.com/fitness/video/3313/korean_chi_therapy

Korean Chi Therapy is based on Taoism or "The Way", the philosophy of Laozi which is thousands of years old. It uses traditional energy channel concepts similar to Chinese medicine but treatment is done with sound energy instead of needles. The process is based on the 360 energy channels in the body, recognizing that when there is restricted energy flow then illness and disease can result.

A normal session has the client fully clothed and face down on a massage table. The therapist's hands move slightly above the body while making special sounds to open the flow of healing energy and channeling life force or chi. There may also be slight fingertip pressure on certain points to open the energy channel if needed. There are seven major life-force frequencies so sounds are made to meet specific needs of each individual.

Learning Korean Chi Therapy also has health benefits. Meditation is part of the learning process for healing sounds so they can learn to open their own three warm-energy centers. There are also slow, gentle movements involved in the training process similar to Tai Chi, a beneficial type of moving meditation.

KOREAN HAND THERAPY or Koryo Hand Therapy (KHT)
http://www.khtsystems.com/sectiona.htm
http://www.koryohandtherapy.com/

Koryo Hand Therapy, also called Korean Hand Acupuncture or Soojichim, is a combination of reflexology and acupuncture for the hand. It's based on the concept that the entire meridian system of the body is represented in miniature in the hands.

The process was developed in the 1970s by Korean acupuncturist Dr. Tae-Woo Yoo, O.M.D., Ph.D. There are believed to be 14 micro-meridians and 345 acupuncture points in each hand which provide energetic access to meridians, body structures and internal organs. These points can be stimulated using needles, metal pellets, small magnets or other devices using massage, heat, colored light, laser or electricity.

There are different types of diagnostic techniques used with KHT including the taking of pulses, abdominal diagnosis and standard medical techniques. Therapies include: Corresponding Point Stimulation; Micromeridian Balancing; Five Element Tonification; Eight Extra Ordinary Points and Special Points Therapy among others.

K.H.T. Systems has been active since 1993 in promoting this process in the U.S. and they offer both correspondence and seminar training including a one-year certification program. There are certification standards being developed in close association with the American Institute of Koryo Hand Therapy.

USER COMMENTS: *"It is with great pleasure that I can inform you that procedure performed last Monday and Wednesday has cured my shoulder/rotor-cuff ailment. I had had severe pains in that shoulder for nearly 1-½ years and you fixed it in just a few minutes. I am amazed at how accurately those pressure points in my hand worked. I had tried massage and even went to the extreme of pain killers to help me get a decent nights rest. Thank you so very much!!!"*

"When my MS pain begins, I wrap my hand around the treatment stimulator and squeeze. I use it on the side that I am currently having pain. I stretch-out my hand, palm up. I set the stimulator in the crease of where the palm meets

the fingers and wrap the fingers around and squeeze. The best part of the stimulator is I can use it in class, meetings or watching TV. No one knows it but me. I get relief in about 10 minutes. Sinus headaches were a huge problem for me and as they begin I get out the stimulator and pain no more. I have used it with muscle pain, MS pain, arthritis pain, joint pain etc."

MAGNETIC THERAPY

www.biomagnetic.org or www.magnetictherapyfacts.org

Magnetic Therapy or Magnet Therapy or Magnotherapy has been around for more than 2,000 years in a variety of civilizations as a method for natural healing and pain relief. It makes use of the static magnetic fields produced by permanent magnets in a variety of products such as bracelets, blankets, shoe insoles and other items. When combined with the reduction of stressful electromagnetic fields it's called **Biomagnetic Therapy**. **Electromagnetic Therapy** or **Magnetobiology** is the use of electromagnetic energy to the body for the treatment of disease.

There are two schools of thought about how this therapy functions in the human body. The first concept is biologically based noting that there are metals like iron in our blood and cells. The use of a magnetic field on a wound or injury simply attracts the metals in our blood in order to increase the flow of oxygen, nutrients, hormones and other healing factors to that location.

The other concept is based on energy medicine and the belief of a life force in the human body that's been called Chi in Traditional Chinese Medicine or Prana in Ayurvedic medicine. It is considered a force of nature similar in some ways to gravity. Illness, injury and disease produce interruptions in the natural flow of this living energy and the use of magnets helps to restore the natural balance of energy. It is believed that our bodies produce negative energy as a normal healing response so a negative pole is frequently used.

Magnetic devices are now registered as medical devices available by prescription in 54 countries around the world while the Food and Drug Administration classifies the application of magnetic fields as "not essentially harmful". There are numerous regulations prohibiting the marketing of magnetic therapy products with the claim of therapeutic effects, especially for serious conditions like cancer and AIDS.

USER COMMENTS: *"As a practitioner it's clear that the evidence over 12 years of experiments demonstrates biomagnetic therapy to be effective for facilitating the natural healing response of the body & accelerating wound healing, pain reduction and resolving inflammation. I have worked with over thousands of clients and everyone benefits who tries. I was a skeptic years ago but now this is my life's work to help others learn the truth about the simple noniatrogentic benefits of biomagnetic therapy."*

POLARITY THERAPY

www.polaritytherapy.org

Polarity Therapy is a comprehensive health system developed by Randolph Stone, D.O., D.C., N.D. based on the human energy field. It involves four elements: energy-based bodywork; diet; exercise and self-awareness. The Polarity model is built on the concept that health is the result of the body's energy system being in its natural state, without blockage or hindrance. It is a blend of science and spirituality working to balance the physical, emotional and spiritual facets of the individual for health and vitality.

Polarity Therapy incorporates many of the features of other energy-based processes including the yin-yang concepts of Traditional Chinese Medicine along with the Three Principles and Five Chakras of Aryuvedic Medicine. Some of the basic principles of Polarity Therapy are:
- The hands are conductors of energy
- Energy can be manipulated by both practitioner and client
- Clients respond to the touch and consciousness of the practitioner
- Clients have a subconscious intelligence and self-regulating capacity

Sessions usually have 60 – 90 minutes of physical and verbal interaction with clients remaining clothed. The practitioner measures the client's energy using palpitation, observation and by through the interview process. Touching the client may have a variety of intensity levels depending on the situation. The practitioner helps the client to develop self-awareness of energetic sensations which are often described as tingling, warmth or a wave-like sensation.

One of the features of Polarity Therapy was described by Dr. Stone as a "fixation at the negative pole" which is the tendency to become attached to events, people, things or experiences which reduces flexibility, adaptability and our ability to forgive.

Born Rudolph Bautsch in Austria in 1890 he moved to America as a child and changed his name in the 1920s. He was a doctor of osteopathy, a chiropractor and a doctor of naturapathy. His first book on Polarity Therapy was published in 1947. He maintained a successful medical practice in Chicago for 50 years using a variety of techniques because his motto was "Whatever works, works!" In the 1960s he began to teach his Polarity Therapy to others.

The American Polarity Therapy Association was founded in 1984. The fourth edition of their Standards for Practice and Education was published in 2003. The Associated Polarity Practitioner (APP) level requires 155 hrs of approved training while the Registered Polarity Practitioner (RPP) level requires 675 hrs of training.

PRANIC HEALING (PH)

www.pranichealing.com

The **Pranic Healing**® system is an energy-based, non-contact healing technique that utilizes "prana" or life force energy to balance, harmonize and transform the body's energy processes. It was developed by Grandmaster Choa Kok Sui to realign the body's entire energy system to promote the body's healing ability. The system is a combination of many different healing techniques including Chinese Chi Kung, Japanese Reiki, the "laying on of hands" from the Christian tradition, Tibetan healing arts and more.

The word "prana" is from Sanskrit and means "life-force". The healing system is based on the principle that the body is designed to repair itself and that the process can be accelerated by increasing the life force energy. Vital energy is added to the body's energy aura without contact so it can absorb and then redistribute it to the organs and glands

Pranic Healers are trained to activate the chakra energy centers in their hands so they can sense the flow of energy in others. Waving and moving their hands back and forth at various distances from the physical body allows them to sense heat, tingling sensations and pressure which are the symptoms of energy flow. Once they are able to scan a person's energy field to locate blockages they learn how to cleanse, energize and revitalize an area with a blockage or restricted flow using new prana to heal physical and emotional imbalances.

Other techniques include **Advanced Pranic Healing**sm which modifies the type of energy used for healing. In the basic process white prana energy from the environment is used but in the advanced form the facilitator's intention and visualization focuses specific colors on the subject to better heal particular problems.

Another type of healing technique is called **Pranic Psychotherapy**sm which involves releasing negative energy associated with emotional issues and problems. Using advanced extraction methods on the affected chakra energy centers it removes emotional traumas, phobias and addictions.

Grandmaster Choa Kok Sui did not claim to be a clairvoyant nor was he born with any healing ability. He was said to be very open minded and has read the ancient teachings on healing extensively. He had taught his process worldwide so people can heal themselves and others.

Training and certification in this process is done by the U.S. Pranic Healing Center at the American Institute of Asian Studies which was founded in 1991. The entry level of Certified Associate Pranic Healer requires approximately six months of training. Since there is no physical contact between Pranic Healer and client there is no massage license needed but there may be other state requirements.

USER COMMENTS: *"In general, after a Pranic Healing treatment I just feel much calmer and balanced. I feel much lighter and I can breathe better. It feels*

like a weight is lifted. It is very subtle and the good feeling kind of creeps up on you. The healer does not touch you, but after a session I have felt like I just came from a SPA. It's pretty amazing. I am an engineer by training and I would never have believed that this kind of healing is possible, unless I was actually able to experience it first hand. Pranic Healing has changed my and my family's life."

Cravings for Ice Cream and Chocolate: "This year Pranic Healing helped me to get rid of my addiction to ice cream and chocolate. I used to eat ice cream and chocolate every day and lots of it. I can still eat ice cream and chocolate, but I do not crave it and I can go days or "forever" without eating either again. This was two months ago and the cravings have not come back. All the free chocolate that is available for me every day at work is no longer a problem for me."

Bumps, Bruises, and Pain (Children): "I use Pranic Healing on my son almost every day. It helps when he hits his little head playing. My four-year old son is very active, and gets hurt frequently. Pranic Healing help relieve the pain in seconds and my son stops crying very fast. When he was two years old he hit his forehead really hard and I had just learned how to do "sweeping". I swept a hundred times and I could not believe what I saw. The big (2 inches wide, and 1/8 inch protruding) red bump on his forehead disappeared right in front of my eyes. "

"A couple of my neighbors know that I am pranic healer so one day one of them called to find out if I was free, so I asked to come over. Her 18-year-old son had his pancreas injured baldy in an accident. He had been given first aid and medications during his 10 days in the hospital but scans showed the mass of fluid near the rupture didn't seem to reduce. They wanted to try pranic healing so I took the photo of the boy and invoked and applied general pranic healing therapy for pancreas and for fluid mass to clear up. I must have given 2 or 3 sessions before the boy started to feel better but his nausea stopped and he began to feel hungry. I continued the protocol for several more 10 sessions. His mom took him for a scan and reports showed that the mass had reduced 90%. He went back to school. After a few more days she called me to inform that he was completely healed and thanked me profusely."

PRAYER THERAPY (PT)

www.prayertherapy.com

According to the 2002 study by the federal government 45% of Americans have used prayer for health reasons. **Prayer Therapy** (PT) is a process of learning how to pray effectively by combining the insights of psychology with the power of prayer. Prayer is important to our lives because each person needs to communicate with his or her God in order to reach their full potential.

Prayer Therapy began with a grant in the 1950s to William R. Parker, Ph.D. from the Religion in Education Foundation to compare the effectiveness of prayer, psychotherapy and a combination of the two processes. *Prayer Can Change Your Life* by Dr. Parker and Elaine St. Johns reports on this research.

Prayer can be words, thoughts or images but they express inspiration, devotion and affirmation. As an alternative to psychotherapy Prayer Therapy is a systematic process of discovering hidden insights and the power of the soul for personal growth. It is based on the belief that every human being has a body, mind and soul and that while changing thinking or behavior can be beneficial, prayer can be a healing tonic for the soul.

Prayer Therapy must be practiced with honesty and love to be effective, which can be very challenging. Honesty is difficult because we all want to support our own perspective because we see it as being in our own best interest. Love is the healing power but it can also be a challenge.

Different methods may be used to progress through stages of development. Prayer Therapy practitioners may be ministers, medical professionals or simply lay people. There are also several books available for self-help with Prayer Therapy.

Today **Amplified Prayer Therapy** (APT) connects the world of prayer with quantum science.

The works of Dr. Masaru Emoto, a Japanese scientist, are often used to support this new approach. His movie *What The Bleep Do We Know* and his book *The True Power of Water* offer evidence that physical items like molecules of water may be affected by the energy of our thoughts, words, feelings, and even our music. This means that our prayers literally have the power not only to change who we are but also to change the world around us.

USER COMMENTS: *"My friends took me to my first Prayer Therapy class. I did not want to go. My friends got a wheel chair, lifted me, in pain, into the chair, rolled me into the Prayer Therapy class and then left. I didn't say a word for the first three classes and when I did talk I expressed anger at my friends for forcing me to have this painful experience. It wasn't long till I realized my downward trip into depression and arthritis pain began the day my ex walked out on me. I used meditation combined with visualization and imaging to do what I found otherwise impossible to do. Of course, I was encouraged, seeing others in my Prayer Therapy group making gains they never dreamed possible either. Once I started expressing my anger without judging myself, I started to be less depressed. When I was really able to forgive my ex and pray for good things to come to him, I got out of that chair and have been walking, a little hobbled, but pain free, ever since."*

"I was a very successful salesman but unhappy with my choice of careers and my marriage situation. I had no experience with religion other than being required to go to church with my mother and brother when I was young. I was quite skeptical when a friend suggested that I might get some help for my unhappiness by attending a Prayer Therapy group. The insights, love and encouragement of my Prayer Therapy group changed my attitude about myself

and life. I went back to school and got my masters and doctorate in psychology. Happily I have been in private practice as psychologist for over 25 years. The meditation type prayer, combined with psychological insights is, dollar for dollar, hour for hour, the most effective catalyst for change that I know of. Prayer Therapy has given me a deep and rewarding appreciation for the spiritual aspect of life."

"I think that what made our Prayer Therapy group so successful was that through the testing we identified the problem below our symptom and made this problem the object of our prayer. As it says in the book of James in the Bible, we were "praying amiss" before. I am now retired, but when I look back on my life, I realize that taking that Prayer Therapy class was the beginning of a whole new positive direction for my life. I thank God often for that life changing experience."

QI GONG or Qigong
www.qi.org or www.nqa.org

Qi Gong (pronounced chee-kung) combines motion and meditation by combining postures, breathing techniques and focused intentions. "Qi" means breath or the energy produced by breathing and "gong" means work or skill so Qigong can mean "breath work" or "skill of attracting vital energy". The practice is said to go back up to 5,000 years in China and is considered part of Traditional Chinese Medicine.

There are an estimated 3,000+ different styles and schools of qigong but the various practices can be classified as a martial art, medical or spiritual practice. All of the styles are based on the belief that the body has an energy field maintained by normal breathing. Qigong unblocks stagnant qi and restores normal energy flow through the body's meridians. Tai Chi is one category of Qigong forms.

In China and around the world today millions of people regularly practice qigong for their health. The gentle, rhythmic movements are reported to reduce stress, build stamina, increase vitality, enhance the body's immune system and improve cardiovascular and respiratory functions. Visualizations are used to enhance the mind-body connection to promote healing. It's practiced by all ages because its slow gentle movements can be adapted for even for the most physically challenged.

Historically it was practiced extensively in Taoist and Buddhist monasteries as part of their martial arts training. It's believe that traditional qigong was based on the belief that certain body movements and mental concentration along with various breathing techniques would balance physical, metabolic and mental functions. Later these practices became standardized, often in connection with the various meditative techniques of religious practices. Over the centuries many new forms of qigong were created and passed down.

Chinese hospitals have officially recognized Medical Qigong treatment as a standard medical technique since 1989. The 2002 U.S. federal government study reported that 0.5% of those surveyed said they'd experienced this modality at one time and 0.3% said they'd used it in the prior year.

USER COMMENTS: *"A woman friend of mine was struggling with a difficult relationship problem and experiencing anxiety attacks. I taught her a simple Qigong exercise to practice for ten minutes each day. The next day, she called to thank me because after just one practice session, she felt centered and grounded for the rest of the day with no anxiety."*

"A friend had to undergo emergency gall bladder surgery. When I visited her a few days later, she was in great distress partly because she was unable to eat or sleep well. I offered to do Qigong on her. The next day the change in her appearance was dramatic. She reported that not only had she slept well, but she was able to eat some solid food that morning and that she "felt human" again."

"A woman asked me to do Qigong on her because an ultrasound test had indicated another cyst on one of her ovaries and she did not want to undergo surgery again. (She had had surgery the previous year on the opposite ovary). I taught her some simple Qigong exercises and told her to visualize the ovary as normal. A few weeks later another ultrasound was done and it showed that the cyst was gone. So she didn't have to have the surgery."

"I had suffered from arsenic poisoning for almost a year, this went undiagnosed from all traditional medical tests. After 11 months I was awakened one morning to realize I was severely ill, and within minutes went into anaphylactic shock ,and transported by ambulance to the ER where once again misdiagnosed. I went into seizures and lost my speech. At this point I was referred to a Chinese medical practitioner. With NAET and Chi gong she was able to bring me to complete health. I personally feel she saved my life."

QUANTUM HEALING
www.healthy.net/scr/interview.asp?Id=167

Quantum Healing uses energy of different levels or frequencies to heal. Based on theories of quantum physics, it capitalizes on different types of energy that exist simultaneously. Quantum physics has long accepted the premise of multiple states of existence, the so-called "Schrödinger's Cat" where something can exist in more than one state at any one time and the act of observation determines its condition. This concept is also the basis for a phenomenon called "entanglement" or as Albert Einstein described it "spooky behavior" where objects remain connected regardless of time and distance.

Healing with this process uses energy from different levels of existence. One option is for the individual to tap into his own levels of energy to change the level that has the problem. By using our individual higher level of intelligence we can produce changes in the mind-body's energy to promote health. Putting it another way, it's using one mode of consciousness (mind) to heal another mode of consciousness (body).

The concept was introduced to America in the book *Quantum Healing: Exploring the Frontiers of Mind/Body Medicine* by Dr. Deepak Chopra more than fifteen years ago. Dr. Chopra is an endocrinologist who's also taught at Tufts and Boston University Medical Schools who became fascinated with the amazing recoveries of patients given a short time to live. In the 1980s he returned to India to learn about Ayurveda (*see Ayurveda listing*). Returning to the U.S. he combined this ancient knowledge with neuroscience and Western medicine to develop a new understanding of the different levels of healing.

QUANTUM TECHNIQUES (QT)

www.quantumtechniques.com/

Quantum Techniques (QT) is a technique of energy medicine to identify and eliminate problems in the body's energy system that are preventing the body from healing itself.

While traditional medicine tends to focus on a single cause of a disease, energy medicine works on a holistic basis. Stress, pathogens, traumas, toxins and a variety of other contributors often work together to cause disease so it's not simply a single issue solution to solve it either. Treating only one facet or symptom of the problem would be ineffective.

Quantum Techniques works to improve the function within the body's energy field. A person may have the correct amount of vitamins and minerals, water, proteins, carbohydrates and other elements in their body but if there is a communication failure within the body then function suffers. Each type of cell has a unique frequency and diseased cells have different frequencies than healthy cells of the same type. Restoring the proper energy frequency removes the barriers so the body can heal itself.

Individuals first use their specific codes and touch the related location on the body while saying the abbreviation and the word it represents to program their body for healing. Afterwards it will be possible to simply read the correct Time Saver Code and the body will know what to do. This technique uses telephone service as its primary method of therapy although additional materials and information is also available on their website. Phone service charges typically run $6.67 to $8.33 per minute but sessions are very short. The initial session may run up to 12 minutes but afterwards an issue may only take four to eight minutes for a corrective code.

The technique was developed by Dr. Stephen Daniel, a psychotherapist and then as a psychologist for 22 years prior to retiring as a psychologist to work in bioenergetic medicine. Twenty-five years of daily migraines led him to develop QT which he says "... has provided more healing in my life than any other modality." Dr. Daniel has been trained in energy processes by Dr. Roger Callahan (*see Callahan Technique*), by Dr. Nambudripad (*see NAET*) and is a conference presenter on the EFT series on chronic illness along with training in other energy medicine techniques.

USER COMMENTS: *"I wanted you to add tremors to the list of things you can heal because mine are completely gone. My head doesn't shake, my hands don't shake, I don't shake on the inside and I can write and other people can actually read it. Again, thank you."*

"Not only have I been horribly depressed this last year, but have been depressed my whole life. Kind of like a low grade fever, it's always present even when I felt pretty good. I am feeling joy in just being alive and am looking forward to how this healing will unfold in the rest of my life. It's difficult to explain to people who don't understand, they are happy for me, but most importantly - I'M HAPPY FOR ME!!! This is such a neat feeling, I'm not quite use to it, but am looking forwarding to this just being normal."

"Your practitioner spent 30 minutes on the phone this morning and I would say she covered more in that time than the medical profession could in 50 years. The session left me speechless. I'm still running around thinking, "How on earth can she pick all that up?" Many thanks and God Bless."

"I have suffered off and on throughout most of my life from acute panic and anxiety attacks. I tried many things then I found an off-shoot of EFT known as Quantum Techniques, and within 24 hours of my first telephone conference with one of their trained practitioners, I knew help was forthcoming. I've now had about 5 conferences via phone and I am NOT the same person I was 90 days ago. I now totally and completely control the attacks and nip them in the bud, without any drugs, just by reading through their "codes", as they refer to them, where you tune in mentally on different pressure points of your meridians, a quantum version of acupuncture or acupressure."

QUANTUM TOUCH® (QT)

www.quantumtouch.com

Quantum Touch® is a hands-on therapy based on the concept that all healing is really self-healing and that the body will naturally choose a healthy frequency. The process was developed by Richard Gordon and popularized in his 1999 book *Quantum Touch, The Power To Heal*. The process can be used by itself or in combination with other therapies.

Quantum Touch® practitioners learn to focus and amplify life force energy through breathing and body awareness. As they develop and maintain a high field of energy around a problem area, the client's body matches the vibration which stimulates their own healing. The breathing techniques are the key to enabling the client to raise their level instead of dragging down the practitioner. Healing with this process can be done with self-healing, on others by direct contact or over long distances.

One of the interesting features of this technique is the ability to move bones into alignment with a light touch. Practitioners don't actually move the bones into alignment - they stimulate the body's healing ability and energy to move them. Proper structural alignment is critical for healthy energy flow in the body.

Training is available by book, video and workshops with certification by Quantum Touch®.

USER COMMENTS *(by permission from website): "My Aunt died of pancreatic cancer. I went to see her a month before she passed away. She was in a great deal of pain and no amount of pain killer could ease her discomfort. She told me that when I worked on her she was able to sleep peacefully for a short period of time after each session."*

A lady had been in the hospital with severe headache pains. She was there for 4 days. Morphine would not help with the pain. They sent her home. I was invited to see her by a friend of hers. I spent one hour with her. Initially she reported her pain level at a 10 but after a one hour session with her using Quantum-Touch healing techniques she reported her pain level had fallen down to a 1.

RADIAC® MEDITATION UNIT

www.baar.com

www.baar.com/Merchant2/merchant.mvc?Screen=PROD&Product_Co de=100

The **Radiac Appliance**, or simply Radiac, is one of the first devices developed for energy medicine. It was created by America's premier intuitive, Edgar Cayce, more than sixty years ago. Often called the "Father of Holistic Medicine", Cayce had an incredible ability for diagnosing illness and disease. He would lie down on a couch with his hands on his stomach and put himself into a self-induced trance where he would answer questions. His answers were called "readings" and more than 8,000 of Cayce's 14,000 readings were about health. Some of these insights go back over 100 years and it's one of the most comprehensive holistic therapy collections in the world.

The Radiac® does not involve batteries or electrical outlets but it does use electric current. It's been called a meditation device, a bio-electric balance, a stress reducer and more. Edgar Cayce said in one of his 1,000 readings on the device "The use of this consistently will be beneficial to the whole of the system." The device is placed in a special plastic container with ice and water and it enhances the flow of energy through the electrodes attached at the wrist and ankle. The flow of energy is designed to restore and balance the body's energy system.

Cayce had strict instructions for the manufacture and use of the product. First of all it could only be made by someone with pure intentions. Second, it can only be used by one person because it becomes tuned to that individual's energy pattern. Edgar Cayce founded the Association for Research and Enlightenment (A.R.E.) in 1931 and today it has approved Baar Products, Inc. (www.baar.com) because they manufacture this device to Cayce's exact intent. Each Radiac® is hand crafted by Bruce Baar, MS, ND.

Radiac® is a registered Trademark with the United States Patent and Trademark Office.

USER COMMENTS of the Baar Radiac: *After my knee surgeries, I never had a good night's rest, even when taking sleeping pills and pain medication. I have even tried hypnosis and other methods. Now, when using the Radiac, I sleep all through the night, instead of waking up 5 to 6 times each night. And instead of feeling sluggish and groggy, I wake up refreshed and have a much better attitude towards starting the day.*

"I am 73 years old and have been using the Radiac since 1980. I find that it heals tension in the body and relaxes the mind, which has improved my memory. Also, I use it for better circulation since I lead a more sedentary life. It is good for arthritis too, of course. Also, using my more alert mind... I am more creative."

"The Radiac Appliance is for real! I have used it on and off for about 3 years now and find that it helps with nervous system disorders.... When used in the evening or nighttime on a regular basis, I find it helps me feel more mentally focused, calm and collected during the day. I agree with Cayce that 'it would be good for everyone'.

Since I was 11 years old, Edgar Cayce has represented truth to me. Through his teachings and readings, I have gained insight into the oneness of life experiences both physiologically and psychologically as the truth have manifested themselves to me. It was not a leap of faith, but a firm belief in Cayce's assertion that the Radiac would be good for everyone that got me started. My experience with the Radiac Appliance has surpassed my expectations and has confirmed my belief that everyone can benefit from it. The flow of energy soothes and heals tension in my body while relaxing my mind thus improving memory, energy and focus. After using it, the closest parallel would be the energized and balanced sense of well being I experience after yoga. Like yoga, the results have had the cumulative effects of allowing for feelings of well being, health in body and mind and a greater connection to the universal oneness in meditation. I would recommend the Radiac Appliance to one and all."

REFLEXOLOGY

www.reflexology.org, www.reflexology-usa.org, www.arcb.net/

Reflexology is based on the concept that the nerves in the feet, hands and out ears correspond to every part of the human body and their stimulation will increase circulation and natural healing while reducing stress. If stepping on a tack can cause pain and trigger the fight-or-flight response then the same pathways can be used to relax and heal the body.

Reflexology was discovered by three doctors in the 20th century. An ear, nose and throat specialist, Dr. William Fitzgerald, introduced his concepts in *Zone Therapy* in 1917 based on the premise the reflex areas on the feet and hands were linked to other areas of the body in the same zone. He described ten long vertical zones in the body. In 1924 Dr. Joe Shelby Riley published his book *Zone Reflex* which added horizontal zones for the first time. Eunice Ingham, a nurse and therapist, refined the process in the 1930s into what is known today as foot reflexology and began to bring it to lay people. In 1957 French doctor Paul Nogier discovered the existence of an inverted reflex map of the body in the outer ear. In the early 1980s Bill Flocco added Ear Reflexology to the field along with the concept of integrating all three types of Reflexology into the same session for maximum effectiveness.

Reflexology encourages the body to heal naturally and helps it to maintain health. Reducing stress is known to improve immune system function and increase energy levels. The process is used primarily on the feet to stimulate the flow of life energy (chi or qi). Treatments usually last for an hour but each client is unique and a course of sessions may be needed. Consistency appears to improve results but the timing will vary by each situation. Some Reflexologists recommend one session each day for six consecutive days while others prefer once each week for six weeks or as long as needed.

As with any therapy if you have any questions or concerns please check with your physician. Your reflexologists may suggest an shorter session if you have certain types of health problems. Please exercise caution during the first trimester of pregnancy. For comfort and greater relaxation you should not have a session less than one hour after meals and immediately after a session you should drink plenty of water. Reflexologists do not diagnose, prescribe or treat for specific illnesses or diseases. Always research the training and certification of a therapist.

National certification for reflexologists is done by the American Reflexology Certification Board. You can also check to be sure that your reflexologist was trained by a school accredited by the American Commission for Accreditation of Reflexology Education and Training (http://www.acaret.org). There are several how-to books and videos available for self help along with products such as reflexology socks which provide zone stimulation of the feet.

User Comments: *"In the past I was used to having a Reflexology session once a week, now for various reasons I'm lucky if I get it once a year. What I've noticed is I had more energy during the time that I was having regular sessions. I also can tell you that it helps with women's issues."*

REIKI

www.reiki.org

Reiki (pronounced ray-key) is a style of Japanese energy work, a technique for stress reduction and relaxation to promote healing. The term is composed of two Japanese words, "rei" meaning God's wisdom or power and "ki" meaning life force or energy.

As with other types of energy work this process is done by moving and waving hands slightly above the individual's body in order to manipulate their ki, or life force energy. Traditional practitioners usually hold each hand position for several minutes before moving to the next location but there are variations in technique. If an individual's energy is low, blocked or hindered in any way they are more like to feel stress and become ill. Higher energy levels produce health and feelings of wellness. Moving the hands allows the Reiki practitioner to add, move and adjust this living energy. Reiki also uses symbols to attract healing energy during the process.

The ability to perform Reiki is transferred to the student during an "attunement" process by a Reiki master. This allows a Reiki student to tap into the unlimited supply of life force energy to improve their health and the health of others.

There are different types of Reiki. The original form was created by Dr. Mikao Usui in Japan during his Isyu Guo training when Reiki energy entered his crown chakra enhancing his healing abilities. Following this experience he could give healing to others without depleting his own life force energy. Many years later he added the Reiki Ideals to add spiritual balance to **Usui Reiki**. For the process to have lasting results, the client must accept responsibility for her or his healing and take an active part in it.

Dr. Chujiro Hayashi received his Reiki Master initiation from Dr. Usui and he went on to open a Reiki clinic in Toyko. He developed the standard hand positions, the system of three degrees and other additions to the Reiki process.

Reiki was considered Japanese, meant only for Japanese, but Mrs. Hawayo Takata was so insistent on learning it after the process cured her that Dr. Hayashi relented and agreed to train her. She returned to Hawaii in 1937 to introduce Reiki to the West. In 1938 Dr. Hayashi initiated her as his thirteenth and final Reiki Master.

Karuna Reiki is another type of Reiki. Karuna is a Sanskrit word meaning taking action to diminish the suffering of others. It's used both in Hinduism and Buddhism. There are four Karuna® I symbols used in this version of Reiki.

Raku Kai Reiki was developed by Arthur Robertson, a student of one of Mrs. Takata's Reiki Masters. The technique incorporates the Tibetan practices of the Hui Yin, the Breath of the Fire Dragon, along with Tibetan symbols. This style is believed to have influenced the creation of **Vajra Reiki**, **Tera Mai Reiki** and other forms.

Reiki training was added to the curriculum of the Center for Spiritual Development in 1989 and in 1991 the name was changed to The Center for Reiki Training. Training is available in a variety of styles including the Usui/Hayashi method as taught by Mrs. Takata combined with a style based on Tibetan shamanism called Raku Kai and traditional Japanese Reiki techniques.

According to the U.S. survey on CAM use in this country 1.1% of those surveyed said they'd used Reiki or some form of energy healing and 0.5% reported they'd used it in the prior year.

There are many different levels of training and proficiency of Reiki instructors and practitioners. Imara® recommends the first question you should ask is "What is your lineage?" because that's one of the first lessons learned in traditional training. If the practitioner has learned "microwave Reiki" as she calls it, they won't be able to answer the question.

USER COMMENTS: *"I really don't know/understand much about Reiki. All I know is that IT WORKS! I've had it done 2-3 times with great results. To me, it's beautiful, almost mystical, because they never touch you with their hands, yet you can feel the penetrating heat and energy emitting from them. Many years ago I was part of a hot air balloon crew and I wrenched my back. I went to a Reiki Master recommended by my sister back home. I could barely walk up the winding staircase to get to his studio but after the one-hour session, I walked down the same spiral staircase with NO PROBLEM and crewed the rest of the week-end! And have never had that deep, sharp pain in my lower back again. My little nephew calls it 'magic hands'".*

(With permission from www.TheWisdomLight.com)

"Dear Imara, Thank you so much for the amazing insight, guidance and compassion you have shown me in our two sessions together last month. I have been doing MUCH better, and am working on the issues that surfaced. My attitude is upbeat and positive, which is bringing about all sorts of wonderful changes. I am much more relaxed about my path now, and am certain all is unfolding as it should. Again, thank you for the wonderful work you have done for me and for my friends."

"I didn't want to believe her. I didn't believe her. But, she was right. I've learned to listen now. It's helped me to change my life for the better."

RESONANCE REPATTERNING™ or Holographic Repatterning®
www.repatterning.org

Resonance Repatterning, formerly called **Holographic Repatterning**, is an energy process to align your frequencies into a coherent pattern in phase with your life. It is based on the concept that every human being is a pulsing field of frequencies. Problems in our lives are simply areas of non-coherence which need to be retuned to the correct frequency in order to resonate with life-enhancing healing.

Chloe Faith Wordsworth developed this process in the early 1990s as a result of her work with tuning forks and color frequencies to balance meridian flow. It's based on principles of the chakra system of India, the five element meridian system of China with new physics and energy psychology. The

Holographic Repatterning Process for Positive Change works with the HR muscle indicator system to identify and transform non-coherent patterns. The process can be done with a trained practitioner in person, by telephone or used as a self-help technique.

Training and certification is through The Holographic Repatterning Association.

User Comments: *"It has been more than 3 years and the quality of my life continues to improve. My tennis improved right away—my peers were really curious! I continued to explore other areas where I felt stuck. I became aware that while I was thriving in some areas of my life, there were many places where I was scared. I became more familiar with the concept of resonance and how old patterns learned during survival times were obsolete. I became more able to live and respond in the present. Before I knew it my husband and I found the house we had been scared to even try to look for. I felt like my new found confidence even resonated for my family, especially, my husband who was discouraged by the housing market and feared change. He has since had the courage to change careers in addition to moving. As a family, we still have life's share of problems and we coping well and finding joy in the sunrise and sunset like never before."*

"Thank you so much for the repatterning. I wanted to give you some feedback. On Tuesday evening I felt so much love in my heart. I was a little kid just feeling free and loving. It was great. Yesterday, I could see men responding to me differently. Today, I must be releasing old stuff because I am irritable and crying a bit. It still amazes me to observe releasing the layers of "stuff"... more evidence that it is working."

SKENAR or S.C.E.N.A.R

www.scenartech.com

S.C.E.N.A.R. is an acronym for Self-Controlling Energy-Neuro Adaptive Regulation which is both a therapy and the advanced medical treatment device. Russian inventor Alexander Karasev based the original design on the TENS machine concept but while the TENS masks pain, Skenar relieves the cause of the pain by using the principles of acupuncture to harness the body's own healing ability. The Russians continued development of the device because it helped to solve the restrictions of weight and volume of medical equipment for space travel. Russia's version of the FDA approved it in 1986 and it is now widely used in Russian hospitals but it was kept a military secret until the 1990s.

The original development group split into two different companies and the research went forward on two different but similar equipment lines called the 97.4 and the 500/600 Scenar series. In the late 1990s Russian-born doctor Zulia Valeyeva-Frost moved to London and obtained the exclusive rights to manufacture and sell the Scenar in the Americas and parts of the UK and

Europe. In 2000, Jerry Tennant, M.D. accepted the position for training Scenar practitioners in America.

The SCENAR device is used by trained therapists to help the body reactivate its self-regulatory mechanism that's been pushed out of balance by accident or disease. Areas of the skin that are connected in some way to stressed or injured tissues or organs will demonstrate abnormal electrical characteristics. The device indicates what the body needs for self-healing and then different signals are used to bring the brain's focus to the area for more rapid healing and pain relief. This self-regulation is achieved by the body's neuropeptides, sometimes called the body's pharmacy, being stimulated into action by the device with proper treatment protocols.

There are several different models on the market today and the SCENAR is certified by the European Common Market's equivalent of the FDA for pain control. In the U.S. the technology is registered with the FDA as a biofeedback device for muscle re-education and relaxation training. Dr. Tennant has several patents pending on his new generation of the technology called the BioModulator. The device is the cornerstone of his comprehensive healing therapy. http://www.tennantinstitute.com

Training is not standardized at this time but the International Scenar Technology Association (ISTA) was founded 2003 to address this issue and others involved in promoting this healing technology.

USER COMMENTS: *"This is a wonderful device! I first ran across it during a training conference in Seattle when some folks from Canada recommended it for a minor injury. There was a clinic there that charged very little for a 30-minute session and my problem healed incredibly fast with the Skenar."*

"I was in a car wreck 6 months ago and have gone to doctor after doctor since then. They all said I was going to be disabled because I couldn't move my neck, had limited motion in my right arm and walked hunched over like I was 90 years old. I was living on narcotic pain killers every day, frequently several times a day. After just one session with the BioModulator I can move my neck, I'm walking erect again and I feel so much better I'd almost have to call it a miracle. As a nurse with two kids in pre-med this technology is a shock and a thrill. I can't wait until my next session to continue healing!"

TAPAS ACUPRESSURE TECHNIQUE (TAT)
www.tat–intl.com

The **Tapas Acupressure Technique** (TAT) is an energy-based technique for healing anxieties, phobias, traumas and other problems. It is based on the concept that our body contains memories just like our brain and that when a trauma happens there is a type of separation involving the person and the event. The TAT process restores wholeness by eliminating the stress of the event.

Traumatic stress is believed to cause a negative energy charge by the person trying to hold off the experience because it's simply too threatening. In many cases the negative effects can build up in the part of the body most involved with the trauma. The TAT process allows the individual to focus on the trauma to reintegrate the experience and eliminate the stress associated with it but without erasing the memory.

TAT first uses **applied kinesiology** (*see listing*) or muscle testing to see if the body is ready to accept changes. The individual then lightly touches four basic points on the head where several acupuncture meridians merge while going through a sequence of thoughts. The touch opens up the flow of energy at points on the inner corners of the eyes, the "third eye" spot between the eyebrows and up slightly and the back of the head. The steps involve thinking about the problem, your reaction to it and then creating an opposite, positive thought in relation to the problem or trauma. Then the individual visualizes the source of the problem being cleared along the traumatic memories being healed. The Mexican Association for Crisis Therapy has used TAT with children after several natural disasters. The process can even be taught to large groups or be used for pets.

Tapas Fleming explains the technique in her book *You Can Heal Now: The Tapas Acupressure Technique*. The process can also be learned from books and DVDs available on her website and at seminars taught by certified TAT trainers. As an energy-based technique with minimum contact most states do not require any licensing but please check the restrictions and requirements in your area.

USER COMMENTS: *"During my first session with TAT, I experienced a long-standing, painful memory dissolve into a feeling peace and acceptance in a matter of minutes. The memory remained, but the tears and painful emotion that usually surfaced the moment I recalled this event, were gone. I knew I had found something really powerful.*

"For me, the clearest demonstration of TAT's value came during a six-month period in which my sister, who is developmentally disabled, underwent 6 surgeries. I used TAT regularly to cope with the concerns, frustrations and stress that I felt and was able to stay in a calm and positive place to support her. I was also able to use TAT with my sister to help her prepare for surgery, release fears, sleep better and stay calm and comfortable. She soon learned a simple way to do TAT for herself and continues to use it regularly with great results."

THERAPEUTIC EURYTHMY (TE)
www.artemisia.net/Athena/eurythmy.htm or www.eurythmy.org

Therapeutic Eurythmy is a holistic, active therapy often used for children with ADD or ADHD. It is also as a beneficial therapy for anyone interested in becoming more healthy using the principles of Eurythmy which means "harmonious rhythm". Developed by Austrian philosopher Rudolf Steiner in 1911,

Eurythmy has been called the "art of visible speech and song" because it gives physical expression to the sounds of speech and music.

The first Waldorf School was founded in 1919 in Stuttgart, Germany and its first students were taught poetry, music and other academic subjects through Eurythmy classes. The faculty noticed the process produced a wonderful sense of well being, improvements in coordination and rhythm along with improving the health of the students.

The basic physical gestures of Eurythmy are connected to the sounds and rhythms of language and music. The gestures representing the shapes and textures of the environment are consonants while vowels are the inner response. The fundamental gestures build into movements for basic human experiences such as joy or sorrow which can be repeated and intensified to stimulate specific organ functions. Once the basics are mastered they can be used in free artistic expression. **Tone Eurythmy** is Eurythmy performed with music while **Speech Eurythmy** is Eurythmy done with spoken texts such as plays or stories.

A patient of Therapeutic Eurythmy normally learns the exercises through two or more sessions per week over a seven-week period. It's used for developmental, learning or behavioral problems with children or adults but not as a therapy for acute or inflammatory conditions.

Four or more years of full-time training is required to become a performing Eurythmist with additional training required to become a teacher.

THERAPEUTIC TOUCH
www.therapeutic-touch.org or www.therapeutictouch.org

Therapeutic Touch has been called a contemporary healing technique drawn from ancient healing practices. It's based on the concepts that people are complex living fields of energy and that the ability to enhance healing in someone else is a natural human ability. However in order to do this a person must have compassion, the interest in learning the process and have the dedication to do the self development necessary.

One of the creators of TT was Dora Kunz, a woman with a highly developed sensitivity who was able to perceive blockages and impeded flow in a patient's energy field. In 1972, she and Dolores Krieger, Phd, RN, her longtime student and colleague, developed Therapeutic Touch (TT) along with a program for teaching the procedures and attitudes necessary. At the time Dr. Krieger was Professor of Nursing at New York University. They began formal training classes at the 130-acre Pumpkin Hollow Farm, a family camp and spiritual retreat center of the Theosophical Society in the foothills of the Berkshires in New York State.

There are four major phases of Therapeutic Touch. The first step is Centering which involves bringing the body, mind and emotions to a focused and quiet state of consciousness. The second stage is Assessing which has the practitioner holding their hands 2 – 6 inches away from the patient while moving from head to the feet in a rhythmical, symmetrical manner. The third step is called Intervention, also known as Clearning or Unruffling, which has the practitioner facilitating the flow of energy in a symmetrical pattern through the patient's field. The final step in the process is Evaluation and Closure. The facilitator uses their professional and intuitive judgment to determine when to end the session.

Today there are summer intensive training sessions at Pumpkin Hollow Farm but the technique is also taught at universities, nursing schools, hospitals and workshops around the world for both health professionals and lay people.

VASTU SHASTRA

www.vastucreations.com

Vastu Shastra is the traditional Indian method of architecture and design for living spaces that harmonize with the forces of the universe. It is based on ancient texts which have been interpreted in various ways over time, usually by region. Although its popularity has decreased in India with the growth of industrial building its influence continues to this day, especially in temple design.

The process harmonizes living space with the flow of energy (prana) so it is similar in concept to Feng Shui but with different details, for example on directions of placement and materials. Vastu Shastra deals with all places of dwelling - from the earth, to buildings, to movable structures (cars) and even furniture. It details the desirable traits for each category, often based on features like the sun's path, magnetic field of the earth, etc. The morning sun is very beneficial so the East is considered a valuable direction.

The body is considered magnetic with the head being the North Pole and the feet the South Pole. Even today in India it is considered beneficial to sleep with the head oriented towards the South. Sleeping the other way is believed to be in conflict with the earth's magnetic field which is harmful.

There are many different types of consultants offering their services in Vastu Shastra so it is wise to check into their training and qualifications.

USER COMMENTS: *"I had a listing that should have sold months before. Cosmetically, it was very desirable and in a good location. The price had been reduced twice, and still, no offers. I called for a consultation and within two weeks, the house sold at the full asking price. Their perspective not only made sense, it worked!"*

"After seeing dramatic results in my personal life as a result of the home consultation, I wanted the skills and knowledge to apply these principles in every aspect of my life. I feel I now have a blueprint, a compass, to accomplish specific results that are reliable and impressive. I am truly grateful."

VEGA TEST METHOD (VRT)

Website: www.naturaltherapycenter.com/vega_allergy_testing
www.vegamed.de/img/pdf/e_br_expert.pdf

The **Vega Test Method** (VRT) is based on the principles of acupuncture but it uses a machine to measure changes in skin conductivity to diagnose health problems because the first sign of an illness is "energetic pathology". Electro-Acupuncture according to Voll (EAV) began in 1953 when German physician Reinholdt Voll developed a complex diagnostic system on the concept that specific acupuncture points corresponded to illness in the specific organs. He added various homeopathic extracts and substances into the circuit to aid in diagnosis and treatment. The process required extensive testing of hundreds of different points.

Other scientists continued to refine the EAV concept down to only sixty points in what was called the Bioelectronic Functions Diagnosis & Therapy (BFD) method. However another German doctor, Helmut W. Schimmel, M.D., D.M.D., further refined the technique in the 1970s to a single acupuncture point by using homeopathic extracts of mammalian organs into this circuit to detect organ abnormalities.

The fundamentals of the Vega Test device are simple: a patient holds a brass connection to the device in one hand while the other probe is pressed to an acupuncture point, usually on the fingers or toes, while a spark generator produces a mild "stress" to establish a baseline measurement. Following calibration a selected extract is placed in the circuit and the measurement is repeated with a drop of 15 scale units or more being considered a positive result.

There are a variety of Vega Test devices on the market today including the Vegacheck, Vega Basis, Vega Expert, Vega Select, Vega MRT, Vega STT, Vega Audiocolour, Vega Si Trans. Each has its own features and benefits but all operate on the same principles. Please remember that all testing is done with homeopathic doses for safety and be sure to ask about the training and qualifications of the person operating the device.

USER COMMENTS: *"Vega testing is a wonderful diagnostic tool in the right hands - I say this as it does take a lot of training to be able to use it and interpret from it correctly. The Vega test device is capable of checking the energies of all parts of the body which reflect their health or disease. It is also possible to check both food and environmental intolerances.*

"The Vegatest Expert also provides Energy Screening - a general overview before the main testing that enables the tester to identify general trends. This includes an assessment of energy distribution in different areas of the body, of areas where the body does not adapt well under stress and of the likely location of blocks to normal function and normal recovery.

"In experienced hands it is quick and non-invasive - a lot of health information can be gathered about the causative factors of the patient's problems in a

short period of time. Personally I have been using the VEGA EXPERT biodermal screening instrument for more than 15 years and I have often thought that if I was to be going to a deserted island as a health practitioner, what equipment I would take with me. Certainly, the most important would be the VEGA EXPERT."

THE YUEN METHOD™

www.yuenmethod.com or www.ChineseEnergeticMethod.com

The **Yuen Method**™ also known as **Chinese Energetic Method** (CEM) is a type of full-spectrum energy healing capable of healing the source of pain whether it is physical, mental, emotional or spiritual. As a 35th generation Grandmaster of Shaolin Tai Mantis Kung-Fu, Dr. Kam Yuen developed his process by blending a lifetime study of martial arts with modern Western knowledge including physiology, anatomy and quantum physics. He is also a structural engineer and Doctor of Chiropractics who is knowledgeable in nutritional therapy and homeopathy.

The Yuen Method™ is a non-invasive healthcare process that does not require clients to change their attitudes or belief systems for it to be effective in eliminating pain. The principle of energy healing is that your body functions like a computer, it is either strong or weak or any issue. Pain is simply a warning light that there is a problem with the energy flow in the body. Practitioners use their own energy to locate the highest frequency of pain since it is what distorts our body image and allows disease to occur.

Energetic corrections are made by the practitioner directing healing energy into the proper level and location producing instantaneous results. The explanation for this effect is that the healing takes place at the quantum level of pure energy where everything is connected to everything else and time is not a barrier. By aligning all levels of consciousness, pain is simply eliminated.

Dr. Yuen is the author of Instant Rejuvenation, Instant Healing and Instant Pain Elimination.

USER COMMENTS: *"I have systemic pain, a lot of anxiety and a nervous disorder. I have a dark cloak of not wanting to exist in life as troubling as it's been for me for so many years. I don't have that anymore. If depression does start to creep in, I just make a correction to eliminate it. I have almost no pain anymore. I was diagnosed with fibromyalgia in 1998 because they don't know what else to call it. But it was chronic pain, horrible pain that was so excruciating that I couldn't dress myself, or even get up off the couch or out of bed. I couldn't sleep through the night. I took homeopathic medications for some time, but not long enough to notice any results. After Yuen Method treatment I noticed immediate effects. The pain has almost completely gone. I still have some pain in the left shoulder and some headaches. I had terrible abdominal problems ever since puberty, which turned into lower back pain and then irritable bowel syndrome and on and on. Now those are gone. It's a great recovery!"*

"I have metastatic cancer and have received all the conventional modes of therapy, i.e. surgery, radiation and chemotherapy. Although effective in prolonging my life, I was constantly tired, weak and easily fatigued. Ever since I have been under the care of Dr. Kam Yuen, I have renewed strength and vigor and a sense of well being that I have not felt in years. Even though I admit to having no real understanding of Energetic healing, I am now a believer and am extremely grateful for my positive outlook and improved quality of life which I directly attribute to Dr. Yuen."

ENERGY CATEGORY SUMMARY

Is your mind reeling from all of the concepts and possibilities in this final category? Even if you consider yourself open-minded you may have discovered new ideas that stretch the boundaries of your universe. If you're new to this world of opportunities you may have found comfort in the ancient traditions of prayer or Traditional Chinese Medicine. In any case the genie is now out of the bottle, and how you think of yourself and your health will never be the same.

A musical analogy for this section might be an orchestra of dog whistles, sounds that we can't hear but energy that is still very real (especially if you're near a dog). When talking with clients I usually call this the "deep end of the pool" because it deals with so many things that we have only started to get a glimpse of today. Even as we progress through exercises capitalizing on this universal spirit, that part of God within, or however you choose to describe it – it produces a sense of awe. Afterwards it can be difficult to explain in terms we can accept, even though we admit the experience.

This is also the best part of the book because it opens the door to the most amazing possibilities! Your health, your life, can be changed for the better in ways that are almost unlimited but which can be a challenge to imagine. Your future holds such incredible possibilities that you should be filled with more joy and hope than ever before.

Chapter 5 - Insurance

Do you remember the old Jack Benny joke about him being robbed? Jack was walking down the street when a robber pulls him into an alley, points a gun at him and shouts "Your money or your life!" Jack rests his tilted head on his hand in his trademark posture, and after a few minutes the robber shouts again "I said your money or your life!" Jack shouts back "I'm thinking! I'm thinking!"

Thinking about insurance coverage and complementary and alternative therapies feels a little bit like the Jack Benny joke. It can be about making tough choices. As patients and consumers we know how medical care has changed in this era of 8-minute appointments under managed care restrictions. Have you ever wondered why don't insurance companies don't seem to want cheaper, more effective treatments?

Could it be they want higher expenses so the states will approve higher premiums so they can make more money on the financial float and their investments. We know they'd rather pay $50,000 for a heart by-pass operation or $10,000 for a heart angioplasty operation than $150 for CAM methods to prevent problems. It looks like these are really financial companies, not companies that care about the health of their customers. How else can you explain their reluctance to save money, lives and improve the quality of life for their customers?

Have you heard of the term "denial management" yet? It's one of the hot buzzwords in the healthcare debate going on today. Insurance companies make it a matter of policy to "deny-deny-deny" claims submitted by doctors and hospitals for any minor infraction. Fact is, it's nearly impossible not to have a problem with every claim because doctors start out having to select the proper code out of 7,000 basic 5-digit codes devised by the American Medical Association in 1966. In addition each insurance company has their own constantly changing menu of codes and instructions like adding "-u5" to an established code to signify the latest update. It's a moving maze of delaying tactics that the insurance companies claim are designed to improve efficiencies and prevent fraudulent billing. The fact is that today this paperwork war is estimated to cost around $20 billion per year, about half from each side, in unnecessary administrative expenses according to a 2004 report by the Center for Information Technology Leadership.

Companies that are self-insured are beginning to realize the fundamental errors of our current system and are experiencing a paradigm shift in their attitudes. They're embracing wellness programs and health screenings because spending a little money up front saves big expenses later. In a 2006 Wall Street Journal article entitled "The Road To Wellness Is Starting At The Office" they reported on a recent survey by Hewitt Associates that found 42% of companies offered some type of health-risk assessment in 2005, up from 29% in 2001. Some companies are even setting up on-site clinics.

Be aware that most insurance companies don't pay for complimentary or alternative therapies because they are classified as experimental or unproven. This is one of the key factors restricting the growth of CAM therapies and it's a chicken-and-egg problem. Because most of these therapies cannot be patented like a drug there is limited profit potential, meaning there are no companies interested in investing millions of dollars for FDA testing. The National Center for Complementary and Alternative Medicine, a division of the National Institutes of Health, is involved with testing and research of these therapies but their budget is small compared to that of America's drug industry. Since NCCAM has only been in existence since 1999 they're still researching the oldest and most accepted therapies. Their research with the Mayo Clinic on the effectiveness of acupuncture for fibromyalgia was completed in 2005. At this rate it will be decades before many of the therapies listed here are evaluated properly.

There are some insurance companies beginning to pay for CAM treatments, usually for acupuncture, massage, chiropractic, biofeedback and naturopathy. Deductibles may also be higher than for regular medical care. A few insurance companies offer a special policy rider for CAM coverage so this may also be an option for you. Your insurance company may also have negotiated discounts with CAM therapy providers for a lower cost. It's best to discuss your coverage with your insurance carrier before beginning any new treatment.

Some of the questions you may want to ask are:

- Do CAM treatments need to be preauthorized or pre-approved?
- In order for coverage do CAM treatments have to be authorized by prescription from a medical doctor?
- Do I need a referral for CAM from my primary care provider?
- Do I have to see only practitioners in your network to be covered?
- What coverage will I have if I use a practitioner out of network?
- Are there limits or restrictions on the number of visits or amount that you'll pay?
- What will my out-of-pocket expenses for CAM treatment be?

Any time you deal with an insurance company it's wise to keep detailed records of every call and contact along with all bills, claims and letters.

You may also want to contact your state's insurance department about coverage since there are many differences in state laws and policies. They may be able to help you find companies that offer better CAM coverage and what their ratings are for performance.

On the other side of the issue there are also questions you should ask any potential CAM provider such as:

- What does the first appointment cost?
- What do follow-up appointments cost?
- How many appointments are normally required?

- Are there additional costs involved such as lab tests, equipment or supplements?
- Do you take insurance?
- What has your experience been dealing with insurance companies?
- Do I file the insurance claim forms or will you take care of it?

If cost is an issue for you perhaps you can also ask if the practitioner offers a time payment option or a sliding fee scale.

If you are denied coverage for CAM treatment there are things that you can do. First of all, know your plan and exactly what it does, and does not, cover. You may also want to check and see if there is simply a clerical error in the coding. Compare the codes submitted on your practitioner's bill with the codes noted in the document from your insurance company. If you feel that your insurance company has made a mistake with your claim you can request a review because they all have a process for appealing denial of coverage. You can even ask your practitioner to support your efforts, for example by preparing a letter to your insurance company. You can even file a complaint with your state's insurance agency regarding the problem.

There are new options to help with CAM expenses like an FSA (Flexible Spending Arrangement) account or an HAS (Health Savings Account). Some employers offer an FSA to help you put aside pretax dollars each pay period for health-related expenses. Some generous employers even make contributions to your account. You would submit receipts for expenses not covered by insurance for reimbursement.

For people who participate in a high-deductible health plan an HAS may be an option. This is another type of tax-exempt account you set up and maintain, although some employers may make contributions too. You're even allowed to invest your HAS monies to earn tax-deductible interest. For more information contact the IRS or check out www.irs.gov to learn more. Also note that beginning in the 2005 tax year the IRS allowed taxpayers to deduct medical expenses for a limited number of CAM services and products. Please check with your tax preparation professional about this option.

In some cases the federal government may help with some of the health expenses for CAM treatments. You'll need to check with each agency to learn about your benefits. Some assistance may be available from the Department of Veterans Affairs, Medicare or Medicaid (depending on your state's guidelines). The National Center for Complementary and Alternative Medicine does not provide financial assistance but it may be possible to participate in a clinical trial for a CAM therapy. To learn more you can visit www.nccam.nih.gov/clinicaltrials

Chapter 6 – Conclusion

Don't you feel a new sense of hope after reading about all of these complementary and alternative therapies? Learning about all of these new and old options should open your eyes to the amazing possibilities that CAM has to offer you for better health and a better life. Millions of people around the world over thousands of years have proven that there are many different ways to *Unbreak Your Health*™ and treat the source of your problems, not just the symptoms.

Almost everyone seems to know someone who's had a successful, even miraculous, experience with some type of complementary or alternative therapy. Once you begin talking with people about these opportunities you'll discover that you're not alone in your search for better health. You're part of a growing percentage of Americans determined to find better answers to their health questions. People may only have whispered about these techniques a few years ago but today the discussions are open and candid for one simple reason – they work, and they work without drugs. Effectiveness is the reason that a majority of Americans have used a complementary or alternative therapy today, even if they frequently come to it when the traditional medical community runs out of options.

We're at the threshold of a new era of health and wellness, almost a Star Trek type of healing. The paradigm shift in medicine to using energy for healing instead of drugs has already started ... very slowly, but the change is underway. We're slowly leaving the world of buggy whips and Newtonian science for the new age of quantum science and holistic health. There will always be those people and organizations that resist change but improvements for the better are inevitable.

The fact is the current U.S. sick-care system isn't working. In 2004, Americans spent $1.9 trillion on healthcare; an amount forecasters predict will rise to $4 trillion by 2015. We're spending over 16% of our nation's economy on healthcare, more than any other country in the world! While we spend over $6,300 per person on medical treatments the U.S. only spends about $1.25 per person, less than 1% of the nation's healthcare budget, to prevent chronic diseases. Our healthcare results reflect our upside-down system and priorities.

World Health Organization research shows that the U.S. ranks 15th out of 25 industrialized countries based on the measurement of different health indicators such as infant mortality. In 2006, the National Scorecard on U.S. Health System Performance showed a similar situation, adding that we have the lowest life expectancy of those same countries after age 60. The January 14, 2007 issue of *Parade* magazine reported that "We rank 30th in life expectancy for women and 28th for men. ... (and) the U.S. position has steadily declined over the last 20 years."

We used to feel that America had the best medical system in the world. While that may not be the situation today the acceptance and legalization of complementary and alternative therapies may be one way to improve our health. It's time to explore all healthcare options today because we have too many people in this country who are sick and tired of being sick and tired.

Many of our doctors are the first to admit that mainstream medicine doesn't have all of the answers today and these are the ones most open to finding new ways to help their patients. They accept that what they don't know far exceeds what they do know. They honestly try to know and understand their patients, even if it takes more than the time allotted by the managed care companies, because they sincerely want to be healers. These will be the leaders in the new world of medicine because they're open to all opportunities. They're interested only in the best possible results for each patient.

There are also doctors who will probably never change their mind that drugs aren't the answer to everything, many of whom accept payments from drug companies. The *New England Journal of Medicine* reported in 2007 that their survey found 95% of doctors get gifts from drug sales representatives. The drug industry spends more than $20 billion per year on marketing nationwide. The *New York Times* reported that in Minnesota alone drug company payments to doctors increased from less than $2 million in 1997 to more than $12 million in 2004. Combined with the massive retail advertising done by the drug companies over the last few years to influence patients it's not surprising that our healthcare system is drug oriented.

Democrats and Republicans may have very different views of the world but both are valid from their point of view. Doctors are trained to see the human body as a bag of chemicals which is why their solutions usually involve drugs. Practitioners of complementary and alternative therapies view the human body as a complete being of mind, body and spirit/energy so they treat holistically. How you choose to "vote" on your healthcare will depend on your perspective and your particular problem but it's important to realize there are options.

This book is about a new beginning, a better way to enjoy a healthy, vibrant life full of joy and vitality. It's about how you can *Unbreak Your Health*™ by finding the source of health problems instead of simply treating symptoms with drugs. YOU have the power to choose! YOU are the one responsible for your body and your life, but you have to become an aggressive patient and fight for yourself. If you want to treat a health problem this book offers many new options. If you want to become healthier to avoid illness this book offers many new possibilities. This book is simply a tool, now it's *your* choice how best to use it to improve your life.

I wish you more health and vitality, more joy and happiness.

—Alan E. Smith

Chapter 7 – Recommendations

"Protecting the public" has been the slogan used to prevent people from learning about healthcare opportunities outside the mainstream for too long. Today more than 90,000 people each year die in hospitals from infections and problems unrelated to their illness or condition. Can you imagine if 90,000 people died every year from one of the subjects in this book? Yet the medical community continues to stand on their pedestal and point a finger at all of the "unsafe" practices that they don't approve of claiming they're so dangerous that no one should be allowed to use them, regardless of how many centuries they've been practiced. They sound like any other type of business trying to protect their market share by any means possible.

My first recommendation is for every American to have the freedom to choose their healthcare. Let the open marketplace of ideas determine what works and what is best. Americans should have the right to take responsibility for their own health, including the right to explore options not approved by the American Medical Association and the pharmaceutical industry. Today there is a grassroots effort to establish health freedom as a right of every person but it will take the public speaking up and becoming involved for this movement to succeed. The National Health Freedom Coalition is leading efforts across the country to enact new laws to give Americans the freedom to choose healthcare. For more information visit their website at www.NationalHealthFreedom.org.

States have a responsibility to their citizens to reject special interests and lobbyists trying to restrict access to complementary and alternative therapies. I'd like to recommend the Minnesota model which requires only that all practitioners register with the state. They make no attempt to limit who can practice in their state. Like any other business, CAM practitioners should be registered so the state can monitor complaints and take action to protect the public if warranted. Clients should be required to sign an informed consent form acknowledging that practitioners are not practicing medicine and are unlicensed. Clients should be aware of the state's complaint procedure too so there is protection for their citizens but without restricting their access to alternatives.

This Freedom To Choose approach is far different than other states where prevention and restriction from access is the standard. One example would be requiring a massage training and license in order to touch a client in *any* way. Another would be requiring a master's degree in psychology to practice CAM therapies that are as different from traditional psychology as a laser is from a wood fire. Limiting new options for health only helps to protect the status quo.

Another way to improve healthcare in this country is to change the current financial reward system by insurance companies and the government. Today doctors make more money as specialists treating problems than in preventing them as general practitioners. A general practitioner, the old-fashioned family doctor, can catch problems early which saves everyone money but these doctors earn about 1/3rd less than their specialist counterparts. This disparity may explain why other industrialized countries spend far less per patient but get similar or superior results. Today only about 1/3rd of the doctors in America are primary care physicians compared to about half in other industrialized countries.

I've referred to the *White House Commission on Complementary and Alternative Medicine Policy, Final Report* (2002) several times. While expressing several concerns they appreciate the challenge and opportunity that CAM presents for our country.

The report understands the need for the federal government to take responsibility for research and promotion of complementary and alternative therapies because of the limited profit potential of these therapies. In America if there isn't a profit incentive there isn't a reason for companies to become involved in complementary and alternative therapies. Whether through changes in the tax code to stimulate private investment or direct government participation, the federal government must take a more active role to capitalize on CAM to improve our nation's health. It will save billions of dollars in our economy so the subject should be a vital part of the national debate on healthcare.

The federal government needs to become a clearinghouse for accurate, useful and easily accessible information on CAM practices and products. Not every device should have to go through a multi-million-dollar FDA testing process in order for the public to learn about it but the FDA continues to try and regulate every facet of CAM while they fail to regulate tobacco, a product that they know kills hundreds of thousands of people every year but with a powerful lobby and political connections.

While standards of safety are needed it must be recognized that by their very nature many of these therapies and devices do not fit neatly into current classifications. In many cases trying to measure and standardize CAM with our current methodology is like trying to put a square peg into a round hole. New results-based standards and methods are needed and this was noted in the federal report.

CAM advertising practices should be truthful and not misleading to the public but with expanded, legalized definitions and descriptions. For example, terms like Energy Medicine need to be accepted to accommodate the new world of complementary and alternative therapies and technologies. Potential customers should have the right to learn about cutting edge concepts as well as ancient traditions.

While I am extremely cautious by nature about the role of big government in anything, I do accept the report's recommendation for the Department of Health and Human Services to play a vital role in developing consumer access to safe CAM practices. Due to the urgency of the healthcare situation in America the federal government should create a new office of CAM to facilitate the integration of these therapies into the country's healthcare system. However, at this time the National Center for Complementary and Alternative Medicine has become the center for the federal government's policies on CAM. As one of the 27 institutes of the National Institutes of Health this gives the established medical community much greater influence over government policies on CAM, to the detriment of everyone interested in alternative health options.

There needs to be increased communication between CAM and traditional medicine to improve their abilities to work together. There are tremendous synergies possible by combining the best of both worlds but today it's like *Men Are From Mars and Women Are From Venus*. There is fear and distrust on both sides and not enough being done to bridge the gap.

There is a lot of talk today about "results-oriented medicine" as a way to bring complementary and alternative therapies into the big tent of healthcare. Perhaps if doctors accept this concept then they'll be able to open their minds to new possibilities and begin to see new ways to help people heal. If results are what really matter to medicine then CAM has much to offer.

Complementary and alternative healing practitioners also need to change their attitudes because many have a limited perspective. Each technique thinks they need to fight for their fair share of business, even going against other practitioners in the same field. This inability to focus on the "big picture" and cooperate has made it easy for entrenched medical practices and products to dominate the debate over healthcare in America and restrict CAM to the fringes of society.

Perhaps with more cooperation CAM practitioners can develop a new system to help people discover complementary and alternative therapies. Right now there is no "general practitioner" for CAM as there is in traditional medicine which makes it challenging for people to find their way into the field. People with health problems literally don't know where to begin today which is one of the reasons I decided to write this book.

These are only a few suggestions on how to improve the health and lives of all Americans. For anything to change people are going to have to speak up and take action. Today there are literally legions of companies with a vested interest in maintaining the current high-cost/low reward system supported by highly-paid armies of lobbyists working at every level of government.

Your voice needs to be heard. Talk with your doctor about complementary and alternative therapy options. Ask questions with your insurance company about CAM coverage. Ask questions of your city government. Talk with you state representative. Bring up the issue with your elected federal representatives. A rising tide of voices calling for change can sweep in a new era of health and wellness for everyone in America.

Resources

I've tried to list a website on each subject in this book to help you start your search for more information. There are also websites that offer a great assortment of information so they're included here as resources for your journey of discovery.

National Center for Complementary and Alternative Medicine (National Institutes of Health)
nccam.nih.gov/

WebMD
www.webmd.com/

American Holistic Health Information Search Services
ahha.org/ahhahis.htm

National Foundation for Alternative Medicine
www.nfam.org

Health Web
healthweb.org/alternative/

Alternative Medicine Foundation
www.amfoundation.org/

Wikipedia
en.wikipedia.org/wiki/Alternative_medicine

To offer a more complete picture of this field resources presenting the other side of the story are listed below.

- Quackwatch: **www.quackwatch.org**
- The Skeptic's Dictionary: **skepdic.com/tialtmed.html**
- Confessions of a Quackbuster: **quackfiles.blogspot.com**
- Skeptic Magazine: **www.skeptic.com/eskeptic**

About the Author

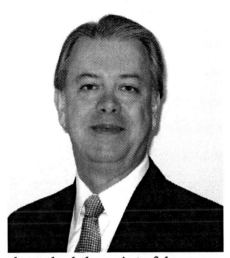

Like many people I only turned to complementary and alternative therapies when mainstream medicine couldn't help me. I reluctantly began my exploration into this new world following a disappointing visit to The Mayo Clinic. It was hard for me to believe that modern medical science didn't have all of the answers, but I was living proof that their knowledge has limits. Being part of the Baby Boomer generation, the group that has changed America at every stage of our life, has its advantages. I knew that the current medical attitude needed to change too. There *had* to be another way to solve this problem, something the doctors weren't telling me. I had reached the point of desperation where I was willing to try, or at least consider, anything. I'm sure many of you can empathize with this feeling.

In one of those wonderful bits of synchronicity in life I read a review of an interesting new book by Bruce Lipton called the *Biology of Belief*. To this day I don't know where I saw it, but I did, and it was the first stepping stone to a new world of hope and health. From Bruce's book I discovered Rob William's PSYCH-K® process and a new way to communicate with my subconscious to discover the real source of some of my health problems.

I took the first PSYCH-K® Basic Workshop and found several tantalizing hints that the source of my health issues was stress caused by the realization that my 20+ year career in supermarket promotions was coming to a close. More than two decades of traveling weekly all across the country had also been physically hard. Because PSYCH-K® is a process best done with two people working with each other my next step was to take my wife to a weekend workshop so she could learn how to use it with me.

My health began to improve and so did my outlook on life. After taking the Advanced Workshop I began doing PSYCH-K® with friends and eventually opened **4 A Great Life** to offer the service to the Dallas/Ft. Worth area. They say that "necessity is the mother of invention" and it's true. I quickly realized that what was needed was a better way to educate the public about all of the wonderful complementary and alternative health options that are available today.

The idea for a new, state-of-the-art reference guide to complementary and alternative therapies was born on April 18th, 2006 with a list of just a few processes. As I researched one process I'd discover one or two more I'd never heard of before, so the list just kept growing. Along the way I've had the privilege to speak with many wonderful people. Their support and their words of encouragement made it possible for me to bring this idea to fruition. I hope that you too will find your way to the right process or device to improve your health and your life.

If you'd like to comment on this book or send your suggestions please visit my website at **www.UnbreakYourHealth.com**

Bibliography

Backstrom, G. & Rubin, B. (1992) *When Muscle Pain Won't Go Away.*

Balch, P. (2000) *Prescription for Nutritional Healing.*

Beck, A., & Burns, D. (1980). *FEELING GOOD: The New Mood Therapy.*

Benson, H. (1975). *Relaxation Response.*

Co, S. (2002) Your Hands Can Heal You

D'Adamo, P. & Whitney, C. (1996) *Eat Right 4 Your Type.*

Craig, G. (Sixth Edition) *The EFT Manual.*

Creagan, E. (2001) *Mayo Clinic On Healthy Aging.*

Gordon, J. (2002). *White House Commission on Complementary and Alternative Medicine Policy – Final Report.*

Hay, L. (1988) *Heal Your Body.*

Khalsa, N. (1991) *Messages From The Body.*

Lipton, B. (2005). *Biology of Belief.*

Moyers, B. (1995). *Healing and the Mind.*

Ornish, D. (1990). *Dr. Dean Ornish's Program For Reversing Heart Disease.*

Renssen, M. (2003) *Meditation & Relaxation.*

Rubin, J. (2003) *PATIENT Heal Thyself*

Sui, C. (1992) *Advanced Pranic Healing.*

Warren, R. (2002) *The Purpose Driven Life.*

Williams, R. (2004) *PSYCH-K, The Missing Piece In Your Life.*

Additional Resources Mentioned

Berard, G. (1992). *Hearing Equals Behavior.*

Canfield, J., & Dwoskin, H. (2003). *The Sedona Method: Your Key To Lasting Happiness, Success, Peace and Emotional Well-Being.*

Chopra, D. (1990). *Quantum Healing: Exploring the Frontiers of Mind/Body Medicine.*

Cousins, N. (1964). *Anatomy of an Illness.*

Emoto, M., & Hosoyamada, N. (2005). *The True Power of Water.*

Feldenkrais, M. (1972). *Awareness through Movement.*

Fleming, T. (1999). *You Can Heal Now: The Tapas Acupressure Technique.*

Groopman, J. (2003). *The Anatomy of Hope.*

Kabat-Zinn, J. (2001). *Full Catastrophe Living .*

Lepore, S., & Smyth, J. (2002). *The Writing Cure: How Expressive Writing Promotes Health and Emotional Well-Being.*

Lewis, S., & Slawson, E. (2002). *Sanctuary: The Path To Consciousness.*

McCabe, E (1988). *Oxygen Therapies: A New Way of Approaching Disease.*

McCabe, E. (2002). *Flood Your Body With Oxygen.*

McFetridge, G., & Pellicer, Z.M. (2006). *The Basic Whole-Hearted Healing Manual.*

Nordenstrom, B. (1983). *Biologically Closed Electrical Circuits.*

Parker, W, & St. Johns, E. (1957). *Prayer Can Change Your Life.*

Pert, C. (1997). *The Molecule of Emotion.*

Silva, J., & Stone, R. (1989). *You the Healer: The World-Famous Silva Method on How To Heal Yourself and Others.*

Tellington-Jones, L. (2006). *The Ultimate Horse Behavior and Training Book.*

Thie, J. (1973). *Touch For Health.*

Tipping, C. (2002). *Radical Forgiveness, Making Room For the Miracle.*

Young, D. (2003). *Raindrop Technique.*

Yuen, K.. (2002) *Instant Healing,* (2003) *Instant Pain Elimination,* (2004) *Instant Rejuvenation.*

Index

Printed in the United States
103071LV00001B/27-30/A